How I Healed My Psoriasis

And You Can Too!

Julie Logan, ND, HbT

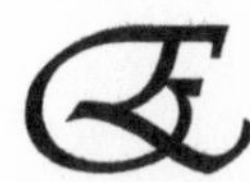

Strategic Book Publishing and Rights Co.

Strategic Book Publishing and Rights Co.
12620 FM 1960, Suite A4-507
Houston, TX 77065
www.sbpra.com

ISBN: 978-1-60976-055-7

Dedicated to my family who always saw the beauty inside me and ignored the skin condition. That is unconditional pure love—thanks.

This book was written to provide you with practical information on how I cured my psoriasis. I have also added further beneficial information to this book. I gained this knowledge while studying to become a qualified naturopath, and have applied it during my subsequent time working in my chosen field. This book is not a substitute for medical expertise or advice. I make no claims to being able to cure or diagnose this disease, or any other. Always seek the advice of a qualified health professional.

The information in this book is the writer's opinion and should not take the place of a health professional.

Do not stop taking any medication prescribed by your doctor or specialist. Before taking any supplements, please consult a doctor or natural health professional to ensure there will be no reaction or interference with your current medications or other health conditions.

Do not start any exercise program without consulting a health professional.

Contents

Section I

How I Got Here

Chapter 1

My Story

It all began when I was about eleven or twelve; the first thing I noticed was that there were small sores on my scalp. After a few weeks they seemed to go away, but that was probably the beginning of it all. I have a memory of my mother asking my grandmother if she had any idea of what they were. At this point, I didn't have lesions anywhere else on my body. In all other aspects I was a normal, fit, and healthy child. The scalp lesions must have gone away, or not caused me too much bother, as I don't have many memories of them until I was a teenager.

When I was about fifteen, I started to get small pink lumps on my skin around my breast area. I visited the doctor, and although he wasn't sure what they were, he said he suspected that they were an allergy or fungal infection, and sent me for a laboratory allergy test and skin scrape. Anyone who has had this procedure done will agree it's not pleasant. Although it was found that I was allergic to cat fur and dust, nothing else unusual showed up.

I returned to the doctor and he gave me a prescription for an ointment, telling me I would probably grow out of whatever was causing the skin condition. For a time the skin did not get any worse, but my scalp became itchy and developed small lesions on it. Once again, my doctor was unsure of what it could be and said I would probably grow out of it.

Time went on and my skin lesions became more widespread, covering most of my torso. Every night I prayed that I would wake to an overnight miracle and they would be gone in the morning, but alas, I didn't get my miracle until much later. Initially, the lesions only had a small scale of skin on top, but over time my scalp and torso lesions developed very large, thick, silvery scales on top of them.

At one point, I had to go to a specialist because my doctor suspected I had a heart murmur. The specialist diagnosed my skin condition as psoriasis. His wife had the same condition and he recognised it. For the first time, my skin condition had a name—not that it did me much good. The specialist also told me that it was incurable, and I would have the condition forever. I was devastated.

For a time I tried some prescription ointments, but I began to believe my doctor and the specialist that there was no cure. I became resigned to having this condition forever. I was lucky to meet the man who would become my husband and the psoriasis didn't seem to bother him too much, although I always hid my skin from him. I was about eighteen at the time, and while I covered my torso, I luckily could still wear skirts and short sleeves.

Later, I had to have a knee operation. By the time the bandages came off six weeks later, I had psoriasis along the length of the incision where they had operated. Within a few weeks I had lesions up and down that leg. Six months later, I had the same operation on the other leg and, again, once the bandages were removed we could see psoriasis lesions around the incision. Now I had to hide more of my body.

Soon the lesions had gone higher up my chest and were progressing further down my arms. I no longer felt I could wear tank tops, or anything else that revealed the lesions on my arms or legs. It was always embarrassing when people asked me what was wrong with my skin, so I felt it was easier to hide it. For much of the year it was easy to hide the skin, but then in summer people would always ask me, "Aren't you hot? Why don't you wear some shorts?" Then I would have to make great explanations to them about my skin. They would always say, "No one will notice, just wear shorts, who cares?" Well, I cared. I cared very much. If I felt disgusted looking at those awful red lesions covered in these thick silver scales, how were other people going to react?

If I did wear something short that showed my lesions, I would spend the whole time thinking that everyone was staring at them and me. As the lesions travelled further up my neck, I found that if I wore anything that revealed them even slightly, or had my hair cut shorter, I would pull my shoulders up in an attempt to hide them. I was always aware of people looking at my lesions as they spoke to me.

Clothes, and what to wear, were becoming a nightmare. It was 1995 and I was getting married the next year, so we went shopping for my dress. Now shopping for a wedding dress is difficult enough, let alone when it has to have long sleeves and a high neck to cover your psoriasis. There were no dresses made that would possibly cover all the lesions. There were many beautiful dresses with low-cut tops and short sleeves, perfect for someone with beautiful skin, not so great for someone trying to hide it. This was one of the worst experiences of my life and my fragile self-esteem was pushed even lower. I cried for days after that trip. We decided to make my dress, which was great, but I was still completely restricted. I felt that I had to cover my skin up, because if I didn't, I imagined everyone saying, "Wasn't the dress lovely? What a shame about her skin!" I wanted (as most of us do) to have a magical wedding day with everything perfect. I prayed and prayed for a miracle; even just for that one day, I prayed that my skin would look normal.

In March 1996, a naturopath set up shop in our town. He had an advertisement in the local newspaper and I phoned him. He explained that I probably had parasites and needed to get my bowel working better. He was an experienced naturopath and I had great faith in him. The most exciting thing was that he was confident there would be a great improvement in my skin before my wedding. For the next eight months I took a lot of supplements and, on average, I was spending between $150-200 per week. Even though he was discounting the supplements and his consultation fee, the costs were still huge, especially when I was only earning $300 a week at the time. Still, I felt it was worth it because I would be free of psoriasis by my wedding.

As the wedding approached it was obvious that my skin was not going to be clear. So, instead of being able to have the wedding dress I had spent my time dreaming about, I had to have the dress that covered my lesions so that I was comfortable. Thankfully, my mother and aunt were fantastic sewers and we were able to make a great dress. It also meant that a stranger didn't have to see my lesions when the dress was being fitted. Sure, I put on a brave face, but sometimes I just cried and cried at not being able to wear what I wanted.

With the wedding and honeymoon done, life continued. I tried all the new creams that the pharmacy and health food shop had, but it was very difficult to put cream all over my body. These creams were often very expensive and in very small containers. I didn't find any of them that made a significant difference or healed the lesions.

My lesions kept multiplying until close to 50 percent of my skin surface was spotted with psoriasis. My torso and back were covered. Every night in bed I would scratch away the thick skin scale on the top of the lesions, with the false thought that it made them thinner. My only bright light was the fact that I didn't have lesions on my face, though I did have them in my eyebrows and in my ears. I would spend a lot of time every morning scratching the scaly top off the lesions in my eyebrows so you couldn't notice them, and then I would pull all the visible skin scales out of my hairline so it wasn't so noticeable.

I didn't wear black because it would show the scale pieces from my scalp. I would have to wipe down chairs after I sat on them, as pieces of skin and scale would be left behind when I got up. I began to have a nervous habit of picking all the pieces of scale out of my hair, leaving piles of scaly skin behind. It was almost compulsive behaviour. Somehow I felt that if I got rid of the scale from the lesions it would make them better somehow.

It was now 1997, I was pregnant with my first child, and during this pregnancy many of my psoriasis lesions began to disappear. My miracle was happening! By the time I had my daughter, about 50 percent of my lesions had disappeared. Unfortunately, I still had lesions over all parts of my body and still couldn't face wearing short sleeves or shorts. I had a couple of very prominent lesions on my neck which were always bright red. Every day I scratched the surface scale off them, thinking this made them look better. All it did was make them look red and angry.

In 2001, I got pregnant again and thought that this would be my saviour. I hoped and prayed that the rest of my psoriasis would disappear during this pregnancy but, alas, this time there was no noticeable change. I wore long sleeves, roll neck jerseys, and long pants. Summer was a nightmare. My self-esteem was in tatters. I was pregnant, fat, and felt very, very ugly.

I pretty much stopped going clothes shopping altogether, because every time I went shopping with someone, I would have to explain that because of my skin I couldn't wear this or that. Instead of a shopping trip being fun, it just made me feel worse. I ended up in tears every time, because I could never find anything that covered my lesions. So even on the hottest summer days, I wore long sleeves and long pants.

During this time of being a stay-at-home mom, I began a diploma program in naturopathy. I decided that I would cure myself! I was studying part time and the program would take six years. In the beginning, I learned a lot about herbs and making herbal ointments. My first mission was to make a balm to cure my own psoriasis. I spent hours researching herbal books, and hours deciding on ways to deliver the herbs to the skin. I learned about the best oils to use for the skin and how they would enhance the herbs. I also found information about essential oils and other ingredients that I added.

Because the psoriasis covered all parts of my body, I decided to concentrate on clearing up the areas that would make life easier. I used the balm on my lower arms and neck so that I could wear a t-shirt during the summer months. I had gained a lot of weight during pregnancy, so my self-esteem was lower than ever and I wasn't too interested in wearing shorts or skirts. So, I cleared up my arms and neck and just plodded along with life, resigning myself to my skin condition. Sure, I could have cleared it all up over time. My balm was successful, but it was messy and a hassle to put on, especially twice a day. It was time consuming, too, and with two kids and a household to run, I just never found the time to be bothered. It all seemed like too much. Perhaps I was just being lazy, or maybe, my self-esteem was just so low I couldn't help myself. I am not sure which, but I felt sure there had to be a better way.

I got caught up in the busy pace of life, raising kids, studying, and everything else that goes hand in hand with modern life. Then my dad was diagnosed with cancer, so for the next few years there was a lot going on. My skin was now the least of my worries. My lesions didn't get better but they didn't get worse either, even with all the added stress.

In October 2007, my son got sick with vomiting, diarrhoea, and high temperatures. Unfortunately, my husband and I caught it too. For the first time in memory, I was so sick I spent the day in bed; I had diarrhoea and vomited once. After my day in bed, I got a cough and sore throat that lasted for a couple of weeks. It just wouldn't go away. At the end of this fortnight my skin began to itch—everywhere! Within another week, there were small psoriasis lesions everywhere, and within a few more weeks I had lesions from head to toe. My skin condition had moved backward ten years in a month.

I fell into a depression. The psoriasis was probably even worse now than it had ever been. I realised that I had probably had a strep infection. Streptococcus infections are known to cause psoriasis (usually in children) and 50 percent of those kids who get it from a streptococcus bacterial infection have psoriasis for life. The lucky other half recover from the condition and it doesn't come back.

I realised that I needed to do something about this. The idea of having to cover my whole body in balm twice a day was a lot of work. Don't get me wrong, my balm is fantastic. It takes away the itch and, over a few weeks of constant use, it gets rid of the lesions. People have had some amazing results with it. It really is very effective when used as directed. The balm is great for small areas, but it doesn't deal with the underlying cause. It just gets rid of the symptom—the psoriasis lesions. I wanted to make sure I got rid of the lesions forever; this meant addressing the cause. I felt sure that something in my body was not working properly and causing the problems.

I searched the Internet and found lots of sites promising cures and instant results, and most of them cost a fortune. I ordered an e-book that looked promising. I paid a hefty sum for it, but figured it would be worth it if it cured my skin problem. Well, this e-book came and I feverishly read it. The miracle cure was to fast on nothing but water! I had paid heaps for a cure that would be impossible for me to do. There was no way I was going to fast on only water for weeks. Sure, it cured his psoriasis, but it came back and he had to cure it again. There must be a better way!

I actually felt ripped off and depressed that my miracle was just another unrealistic cure that I couldn't do. The advertising for the book didn't mention anything about starving yourself; they made it sound easy. There is nothing easy in starving yourself, surviving for weeks on only water, and having to slowly reintroduce foods so the body gets used to eating again. It seemed like the complete opposite of easy to me.

As my naturopathic training was progressing, I was learning a great deal about possible causes and things that I could use to try to cure this condition. I had a conversation with a friend, and she told me that a relative of hers used red clover capsules to get rid of psoriasis. So, I went to work and started to do more research. By now, I was a natural therapist and had established accounts with companies who had herbal products. I found a combination containing red clover, prickly ash, buckthorn, sarsaparilla, burdock, liquorice, barberry, echinacea, cascara sagrada, sheep sorrel, and rosemary. The blend looked great and, on further research of the ingredients, I found it had many ingredients that have been traditionally used for the treatment of psoriasis. In fact, I had used a lot of the ingredients in my balm. I got them to send me the technical data, so I could see what its recommended use and dosage rates were. After more research, I ordered some and started my journey back from psoriasis.

I began taking the capsules, and after only two weeks I could see that the layers of scaly skin on top were reducing. A couple of weeks later, some of the lesions had no scales and the redness had disappeared. Then I noticed that the middle of the lesions had become whitish and looked like normal skin, almost as if they were healing from the centre out. Within two months my lesions had healed up completely. It was amazing! In most places there was absolutely no sign that they were ever there. Some areas of my torso were whiter than others, because they hadn't been exposed to the sun for a long time, but summer took care of that. There were areas where the lesions lingered, but those were the places that had been covered with them for the longest time. I think I will always be at risk of another outbreak, if I don't keep an eye on my body and what's going on with it.

Psoriasis took a lot from me. It took my self-esteem (which I am rebuilding now). I missed out on doing so many things because of this terrible skin condition. It is now that I realise how much it took from me, and as summer approaches again, I am sure I am going to realise how much I had missed out on for all of those years—but not anymore. This is the reason that I have written this book. I want other people to be freed from their psoriasis prison just as I was.

In summer 2008, I went swimming for the first time since I was sixteen. Over nineteen years without enjoying a favourite activity was far too long. The freedom I felt at being able to swim with my children was indescribable. For the first time in many, many years, I enjoyed summer. It was great. I was able to wear a tank top for the first time in years, and I didn't have to cover up when visitors arrived. The sense of freedom was absolutely incredible.

I know how devastating this disease is. I know how much it depletes your self-esteem, how much it can restrict your life and freedom. I have written my experiences here to help others break free from this horrible affliction.

As well as providing you with information about all the things I used to heal my psoriasis, I have added some other remedies, suggestions, and things that may help speed up your progress. These have come from the significant amount of knowledge I have gained during my time as a naturopath. Every system in the body restores itself at a different rate. Every person will have different factors contributing to their condition, and everyone will need a different combination of supplements. Each of you will have had psoriasis for varying amounts of time; therefore, the amount of time before your psoriasis clears up will be different.

I have attempted to keep this simple and not get too technical, overloading you with information. However, I do want to educate you about how to help your body run better.

I want you to be free of psoriasis, too. I know this is a life-altering condition that affects everything for the sufferer, so please read this entire book. I know you will want to skip straight to the good bits, but it is important that you understand that there may be several factors contributing to your psoriasis and, therefore, you may have to do several of the things I have suggested. I want you to understand how this condition came about and the probable contributing factors, so that you will understand the importance of following my advice and adhering to the diet and lifestyle changes.

Hardest of all, you will have to have patience. This condition took a while to take hold, and it may take a while to for it to get better. Your body has been using your skin as a channel of elimination, and it's going to take some time for it to change this pattern. Keep at the new routine, don't give up, the changes will happen. You *can* feel better, feel healthier, and have fantastic skin.

To track the progress of your skin you can take pictures, because sometimes things change slowly and we don't notice the differences. My advice, however, is to only take pictures every two or three weeks, and remember that the healing occurs at the bottom levels of the skin, so you won't be able to see the changes until those layers reach the surface.

I recommend you spend at least three months on this regime and assess the improvement then. I know that we live in a world where we want instant cures, but unfortunately with this condition there may not be one. Don't give up because you don't see results instantly, or even in the first few weeks. The healing will be happening below the surface. What you see on top is the old cells that haven't changed yet. Give it some time.

I know that you are probably afraid to believe that you can beat this condition, afraid to get your hopes up. I understand and have been in the same place you are right now. Just give it a go, make a decision that you will change your lifestyle and diet, and take the supplements for three months. Take one day at a time and watch the changes happen.

SECTION 2

About Psoriasis

Chapter 2

Types of Psoriasis

There are many types of psoriasis; plaque, flexural, guttate, pustular, psoriatic arthritis, and erythrodermic, to name the main ones, but there are others. Psoriasis has been around for a very long time; in fact, even the Bible identified the condition. Although this infliction has a long history, there is so much conflicting information about the different types and what causes it, that it's become a complex condition, with a wide range of treatments available to treat it.

Originally, I believe that I had plaque psoriasis, but there was no dermatologist in our area to confirm that, and I never had a complete medical diagnosis to determine which type I had. I know that in 2007 I contracted a streptococcus bacterial throat infection and, as a result, I developed guttate psoriasis. For me, it was never important to know what type of psoriasis it was—I just had to get rid of it.

You may or may not have been diagnosed with a certain type of psoriasis. It doesn't matter which type you have. I believe the underlying cause is similar in all types of psoriasis. A search of pictures on the Internet will probably help you recognise which one you have. Here is a bit about the different types.

Plaque Psoriasis

Plaque psoriasis is the most common type, with 80 to 90 percent of those affected with the condition falling into this category. It is also known as psoriasis vulgaris. Plaque psoriasis can be easily recognised by its raised, red scaly patches. It is usual to see these patches on the elbows, scalp, knees, chest, nails, and lower back. The size varies from as small as your fingernail to as large as a small dinner plate. This type of psoriasis may or may not itch; it will, however, have thick, silvery scales.

Guttate Psoriasis

Guttate psoriasis often appears after a throat infection caused by the streptococcus bacteria. It is usual to get this during childhood or adolescence. It is characterised by the sudden appearance of very small patches which spread to cover large areas of the body. Lesions typically cover the upper body, legs, arms, and scalp.

Flexural Psoriasis

Flexural psoriasis is also called skin fold, inverse, or genital psoriasis, because it often occurs in the folds of the skin. It may be concentrated in the genital area, under the breasts, and under the armpits. This type of psoriasis is common in those sufferers who are overweight. It is characterised by increased sensitivity to sweating and friction.

Erythrodermic Psoriasis

Erythrodermic psoriasis is also known as exfoliative psoriasis, which covers almost the entire body. It is usually very red, scaly, itchy, and painful. This can be a very serious condition, as it may inhibit the body's ability to control its temperature.

Pustular Psoriasis

This form is rarer than the other types. It usually appears on the palms of the hands and soles of the feet. It can, however, appear in other areas of the body as well. Pustular psoriasis can be very painful, as the skin becomes red and swollen with small pus-filled pimples. Eventually, the pimples dry to form brown dots. A general ill feeling and a fever may accompany this form of psoriasis. Some of the things that may cause this type include infections, certain medications, and sunburn.

Psoriatic Arthritis

Psoriatic arthritis is a condition related to the joints. It will sometimes manifest itself as a skin condition and, at other times, as a joint condition where the joints are inflamed. Usually, these very different symptoms are present at different times. The joint inflammation usually occurs in the hands, feet, ankles, and knees, which become hot, red, stiff, swollen, and painful. Some pain and stiffness can also appear in the lower back, buttocks, neck, and shoulders. This condition can also manifest in the fingernails and toenails, where they may become pitted and develop ridges.

Chapter 3

Who Has Psoriasis?

You are certainly not alone in this condition. Psoriasis is more common than you ever imagined, so don't feel alone. There are many online support networks available, where you can chat with other people who are suffering from this condition.

Psoriasis is prevalent throughout the world. According to the National Institute of Health (NIH), as many as 7.5 million Americans (approximately 2.2 percent of the population) have psoriasis. It is estimated that 125 million people worldwide (2 to 3 percent of the total population) suffer from the condition.[1]

Interestingly, the only group of people who seem to have no incidence of psoriasis are the Aborigines in Australia. There doesn't seem to be a clear indication of why this is. I suspect that their traditional diet keeps their livers, kidneys, and bowels working well.

Two percent of the UK population suffer from a form of psoriasis which is visibly apparent. Five percent have psoriasis which is detectable upon close inspection of the skin. It is found in all races, but is often more apparent in cultures with less sun exposure.[2]

---

1 "Statistics," National Psoriasis Foundation, http://www.psoriasis.org/netcommunity/learn_statistics

2 Natural Organic Health website, "Psoriasis, Conventional Medical Treatment," http:// http://www.health-report.co.uk/psoriasis_medical_view.html

I suspect most sufferers of psoriasis are miserable; I know that I was. In fact, in some countries psoriasis makes you eligible for a government benefit, as it is seen as a debilitating disease that sometimes prevents people from working. Some countries have specialised hospital wards set up for psoriasis sufferers where they paint harsh chemicals onto the lesions in an attempt to cure them. While this can be effective, the lesions often return in a year or so. Personally, I'm not a fan of putting harsh chemicals on my body.

I wanted to create a treatment protocol that supported overall health, not create more problems in other areas of the body. There are many medications being used to treat psoriasis, including some chemotherapy drugs. Some of these drugs have significant side effects. I am not here to run any other treatment down. I am not a doctor and don't understand their treatment protocols, just as they probably don't understand mine. I am not here to say their way is wrong and my way is right. I simply want to educate you from the point of view of a fellow sufferer who is now free from the disease, and to provide you with some options that I have found very effective, in the hope that you will be released from your psoriasis prison as I was.

Chapter 4

What Creates Psoriasis?

There are many conflicting ideas and research about the possible causes of psoriasis. Some say it is caused by an immune deficiency, while some suggest that it is genetic. I had a great grandmother who had psoriasis (I am not sure what type) and a cousin who had an occurrence of pustular psoriasis that came and went. No other close blood relatives that I know of have had it. There are suggestions that stress may cause it, or make it worse. I didn't notice that it got worse, but others see a difference when they are under stress. My psoriasis generally didn't itch. The only time I had the itch was when it was coming back after my streptococcus infection, but once the lesions erupted the itch stopped. For others, the itch almost drives them crazy.

Through my experience, naturopathic training, and subsequent work, I have my own theories about psoriasis and its cause. I believe that it's a symptom of an overloaded system, one loaded with toxins because it is not eliminating them properly, due to the malfunction of the normal elimination channels. When the internal elimination systems are not working, the body will eliminate unwanted nasties through any means necessary. The skin is a large elimination channel, and I believe when the body uses it to eliminate toxins and waste, it causes skin conditions, including psoriasis.

There can be many reasons why the elimination systems are not working properly. Our modern diets contain lots of sugar, preservatives, chemicals, and colourings, and are lacking in pure water, fibre, and nutrients. These types of diets lead to constipation, a gut bacteria imbalance, digestive problems, liver function decrease, and general overloading of the body.

Whilst I believe that the main factor is faulty elimination, there are many factors that contribute to this condition. For example, vitamin or mineral deficiencies, digestive problems/dysfunctions, constipation, bowel bacteria imbalance, food allergies/intolerances, environmental toxins, liver dysfunction, and dehydration, can all play a part. All of these issues need to be looked at and resolved wherever possible, for you to have the best chance of getting rid of your psoriasis.

Section 3

Contributing Factors in Psoriasis

Chapter 5

Modern Foods and Diets

Fairly simply, I believe that we are putting things into our bodies that are non-digestible or recognisable and our bodies are having difficulty neutralising, processing, and eliminating them, as well as trouble absorbing important nutrients. Take notice of all the artificial ingredients in your foods. To make manufacturing and storage easier, many potentially harmful additives are often put in our foods.

We demand that our food remains unspoilt for longer, so preservatives are added to lengthen the shelf life. We like food to look great, so the producers add colourings and other ingredients to make our food look inviting. The growers also use a huge number of sprays and pesticides on our fruits and vegetables to stop them from being damaged by fungus and pests. These chemicals seep into the produce we are eating and, therefore, enter our bodies. Some of them are sprayed with chemicals to make them grow faster or bigger. We demand fruit out of season, and from other countries, so they are often picked early before their full nutrients have developed, put in cold storage, and shipped. Some are kept in cold storage for six months or more, and I believe that most nutrients are gone from them after that length of time. Produce imported into countries are often sprayed with more dangerous chemicals to reduce the risk of transferring pests, and ensure that they do not begin to spoil.

We live in a society that demands we work more and, therefore, we spend less time preparing our own meals. The result is people are eating more processed, less nutritious foods. Most fast foods have little or no vegetables, the ingredients are highly processed, and the cooking methods often increase the saturated (bad) fats, therefore increasing our cholesterol levels and causing further health problems. A lot of convenience foods are high in calories; some meals may contain over 50 percent of your daily calorie needs in one meal. Sugar and sodium levels are often too high, giving us a taste for excessively sweet or salty foods. I am not saying fast foods have no nutritional qualities, but their nutritional value is usually limited, and they often contain artificial ingredients and processing agents that can be quite toxic to the body.

Frozen vegetables, and some fruits, can be highly nutritional and have the bonus of being convenient. Vegetables are often picked and frozen within a few hours, and contain as much nutrient content frozen as they do fresh. Just ensure they do not contain any additives, salt, sauces, or chemicals. Use them within three months of buying, or by their use-by date, to ensure maximum nutrient content.

Processed foods are very convenient and tasty but are produced to sell, not to provide nutrition. Processed foods contain a myriad of ingredients like flavour enhancers, emulsifiers, synthetic colourings, bulking agents, bleaching agents, antioxidants, artificial sweeteners, anti-foaming agents, enzymes, flavours, foaming agents, food acids, glazing agents, humectants, minerals, mineral salts, preservatives, propellants, raising agents, stabilisers, thickeners, vegetable gums, and vitamins, to name just some.

The other problem is the lack of nutrients in a lot of processed foods. White flour has the outer germ and bran removed, to produce lighter, finer cakes and baked goods, and this germ and bran may contain many of the nutrients. White flour still contains nutrients, but in a smaller amount compared to whole wheat flour.

Let's compare the nutrient values between whole wheat flour and unenriched, white flour. The information in the following table is from 2007 from the U.S. Department of Agriculture's Agricultural Research Service. The figures are based on one hundred grams, or three ounces, of flour. As you will see on this table, there is a significant reduction of nutrients in the all-purpose flour, especially the amount of dietary fibre.[3]

Nutrient	Whole Wheat Flour	All-Purpose Flour
Total Dietary Fiber	12.2g	2.7g
Calcium	25mg	15mg
Iron	3.6mg	1.2mg
Magnesium	124mg	22mg
Phosphorus	332mg	108mg
Potassium	340mg	107mg
Zinc	2.8mg	0.7mg
Copper	0.4mg	0.1mg
Manganese	4.1mg	0.7mg
Selenium	70.7mg	33.9mg
Thiamine	0.5mg	0.1mg
Riboflavin	0.1mg	0.04mg
Niacin	5.7mg	1.3mg
Pantothenic Acid	0.9mg	0.4mg
Vitamin B6	0.3mg	0.04mg
Folate	43mcg	26mcg
Vitamin E	1mg	0.06mg
Total Fats	1.9g	0.98mg

3 "USDA National Nutrient Database for Standard Reference, Release 21," USDA website, http://www.ars.usda.gov/nutrientdata

Chapter 6

Deficiencies

Because many psoriasis sufferers do not digest their food properly, they are also not assimilating adequate nutrients from their food. The body is constantly trying to maintain balance. If you intake too much of one mineral or component, your body may have to use up other minerals or components to adjust the balance. As much of our food-producing land has been used many times over in a lot of areas, there are often fewer nutrients in the soil; therefore, the food produced on this land contains fewer minerals than it did one hundred years ago.

There can be many factors that cause a deficiency, including having too much of a certain mineral in your body. You can receive minerals from sources other than just food. Copper water piping was commonly used from about 1940. Those pipes in your house may cause you to have excessive amounts of copper in your body, which will reduce the amounts of zinc and manganese in your system, as these nutrients are used to process copper. There is always a delicate balance in your body between all the necessary nutrients.

You may have a good diet, but your problems may have started at birth from the deficiencies that your mother had. Also, as a child you ate what your parents or caregivers made for you and, therefore, may have developed similar tastes and likes, perhaps carrying on this deficiency trend due to your dietary intake and the types of food you typically eat.

Diet is not the only cause of nutritional deficiencies. Lifestyle or work environments cause you to burn up large amounts of nutrients, processing and eliminating the chemicals you come in contact with. For instance, perhaps you work in a very stressful job. Stress is known to burn through the B-group vitamins.

Zinc Deficiency

Although a deficiency in many nutrients may play a role in psoriasis, one very significant mineral deficiency, zinc, can be a direct contributor to it.

Zinc is a vital nutrient. It helps with the absorption of other nutrients, as well as being a catalyst in over a one hundred actions in the body. Zinc is needed for growth and development, mental stability and calmness, and the development and health of sex and fertility organs, including prostate health. Zinc is vital in wound healing and skin health. It helps regulate cholesterol in the body, assists hair growth, helps regulate other minerals in the body, helps eliminate toxic metals such as copper and lead, and is required for healthy muscle, liver, kidney, and eye tissues.

Signs of zinc deficiency

Zinc deficiency can cause the following symptoms:

- stunted growth
- impotence
- infertility
- enlarged prostate
- PMT—premenstrual tension
- poor learning abilities
- stress
- anxiety
- depression
- lowered immune function

- slow healing of wounds
- acne
- psoriasis
- loss of taste and sense of smell
- diabetes
- high cholesterol
- heart problems
- high blood pressure
- photophobia (intolerance to light)
- white spots on nails

Whole food sources of zinc include: carrots, tomatoes, corn, broccoli, silver beet (chard), kale, green beans, peas, onions, beetroot, potatoes, pumpkin, mushrooms, olives, apples, peaches, apricots, bananas, paw paw, pineapple, beef, lamb, pork, liver, chicken, turkey, oysters, clams, shrimps, crab, sardines, milk, cheese, eggs, peanuts, hazelnuts, sunflower seeds, wheat, rye, oats, brown rice, and parsley.

Before you begin taking a zinc supplement, I recommend you get tested. Taking supplements when you do not need them can cause as many problems as a deficiency. An easy zinc taste test can be done to assess your level. A 10ml liquid zinc solution is put into the mouth for ten seconds, then swallowed or spat out. The resulting taste will indicate the level of your deficiency, whether you will need liquid zinc supplementation, or if zinc tablets will be sufficient. Often, health food shops and pharmacies will provide this test free of charge. When you have a significant zinc deficiency, supplementation will be necessary to build your levels back up. Once you have a deficiency, you may not be able to eat zinc-rich foods in large enough quantities to rebuild your zinc stores. Supplements will be your best way to get your levels back up in the smallest amount of time. Once you get your level restored, you should be able to maintain the balance by eating zinc-rich foods or taking a balanced vitamin/mineral supplement.

Chapter 7

Digestion

Digestion is an important factor in psoriasis. There is a lot of information to suggest that people with psoriasis do not absorb adequate nutrients from their food. When you do not digest and assimilate nutrients from your food, your body will show many symptoms. Let's look at how the digestive system works; this will help you to understand the importance of good digestion.

The Digestive System

The digestive system has two parts. The first part is the tubing (gastrointestinal, or GI, tract) that extends from the mouth to the anus. The GI tract transports the food through the body and digestive process, using a process called peristalsis, which is a wave-like contraction of the muscular wall of the tract. This breaks down the food by churning and moving it. The second part involves the organs that aid in the digestion process, which include the teeth, tongue, saliva glands, liver, gallbladder, and pancreas. Except for the teeth and tongue, these other organs break down the food particles chemically.

Let's take a journey down the gastrointestinal tract. Digestion begins in the mouth. Chewing initially breaks down food into smaller pieces. The tongue mixes it around and helps to break it down further. Often, this can be the very place where your problem starts. People do not always allow adequate time to eat and barely chew their food in their haste to get through the meal. This means that their food is not able to be digested properly, because the particles are too big.

Take the time to sit down and eat. Chew your food well before swallowing.

Chewing is only part of the digestive process that happens in your mouth. As you chew your food, saliva is released into your mouth. Saliva has several jobs. It helps lubricate the food to allow it to slide easily down the GI tract; it also begins dissolving it, as it contains enzymes that start the chemical breakdown. Also, as you chew it triggers the release of digestive juices in your stomach. By chewing food adequately, you allow more time for the digestive juices to be released before the food arrives in the stomach.

Once you swallow, the food transfers into the stomach. The absorption of nutrients does not happen in the stomach. Instead, it mixes the food with digestives juices, stores it until it begins to break down, then it sends it on its way.

The food then travels into the small intestine, which triggers the liver and gallbladder to deliver bile, and the pancreas to deliver enzymes. The liver produces bile for the absorption of fats and to chemically break down amino acids. It is also a storage house for vitamins and minerals. The liver is also responsible for detoxifying the body of drugs and chemicals. The gallbladder is attached to the liver by a small duct. The gallbladder stores the bile produced by the liver and releases it into the small intestine when needed. The pancreas secretes pancreatic juices into a small tube connecting the stomach to the small intestine. This fluid neutralises the stomach acid and contains digestive enzymes that break down proteins, fats, and carbohydrates. The pancreas also has another very important role. It produces insulin and other hormones that maintain blood-sugar levels.

The small intestine is the main area for the absorption of nutrients.

Finger-like tissues called villi line the small intestine and increase the absorption area. The villi absorb nutrients, and secrete enzymes necessary for digestion. The small intestine also contains beneficial bacteria that also aids in digestion. The necessary good bacteria in the small intestine are called lactobacillus.

Food is then transferred into the large intestine. The large intestine also houses beneficial bacteria called bifidobacterium. These bacteria eliminate toxic bile by-products, convert unabsorbed carbohydrates into absorbable organic acids, and are involved in the metabolism of lipids. Even a minor imbalance of these bacteria can cause many uncomfortable symptoms, but worse than that, can cause serious nutritional deficiencies. The large intestine is the place where fermentation of soluble fibre and undigested carbohydrates occurs. Another important role of the large intestine is to absorb water.

A lot of processes occur in the digestive system, so it is vital that it be kept as healthy as possible for you to maintain good health. Take notice of how well your digestive system is working, and any symptoms you may be having. Do not skip the dietary changes I suggest. These changes may be crucial to ensure your digestive system is working correctly and your body is receiving adequate nutrients.

Chapter 8

Constipation and Bowel Health

Constipation is a subject that is often not talked about, even though there are many people who believe that death begins in the bowel. Every system in your body will be affected if your bowel is not working correctly; you will be poisoning yourself from within, and your body will not be receiving adequate nutrients from your food. I know that this is an uncomfortable and taboo subject, but it is a vital one for the healing of your psoriasis.

Many psoriasis suffers have constipation or bowel problems. My definition of constipation is having less than one bowel movement every day. In fact, I believe that you should have three every day, especially since most people eat three meals per day. On the other hand, do not be fooled that because you are having a bowel motion every day that your digestive system is healthy. Take notice of the following categories and types of bowel movements, and what they may be signalling about your digestive health.

A lot of people do not realise that their bowel movement is abnormal, until they are educated about what a healthy motion should be like. I know that not everyone likes to talk about their bowel movements, but it is usually the first thing I discuss with my clients because it holds vital information. I hope that you do not skip this chapter just because it makes you uncomfortable.

It is vital that you realise what is healthy and what is not, so that you can monitor your bowel health yourself. Bowel health is of great importance; it is the powerhouse of the whole body. If your bowel isn't working properly it will affect every other organ system and its ability to function well.

For a more in-depth understanding of bowel health I recommend that you read *Tissue Cleansing Through Bowel Management* by Bernard Jensen. It contains a wealth of information about cleansing the bowel and maintaining its health.

Healthy Faeces

What should healthy faeces look like? A healthy diet and healthy gastrointestinal tract should produce a bowel motion that is usually medium brown in colour, well formed, odourless, and easy to expel.

If your bowel movements are not like this then you have some work to do. Here are some common types of unhealthy faeces, and possible reasons why they may be occurring. This list is not complete, and it is not intended to diagnose any associated conditions. It is only a guide to show you that changes to your diet are necessary. If you are concerned about your bowel health, please visit your doctor or health professional and get it checked.

Floating faeces

If your faeces float it could be a sign of poor absorption of nutrients and excessive gas. Usually, this is diet related.

Sticky faeces

A normal bowel movement usually contains about 1 percent fat. Faeces that stick to the toilet bowl, and are soft and very smelly are usually called steatorrhoea. They typically contain about 7 percent fat. This type of faeces usually indicates there is a problem with the body's ability to break down fat adequately. The problem could lie in the pancreas not producing adequate enzymes to break it down, or the small intestine may not be absorbing the fat properly. If you only have this type of stool occasionally, it can be caused a meal very high in fat the day before. If this kind of bowel movement is common for you, please have it checked by your doctor.

Hard faeces

Hard faeces can indicate constipation, constant dehydration, a low-fibre diet, or one high in sugar and white flour products. It may also indicate lack of exercise or presence of parasites, but can also be caused by not defecating when you get the urge, because the stool is sitting in the bowel for longer than it should and is drying out. Usually these hard faeces come out in little pieces and are difficult to expel, leaving you still feeling full, even after you have tried hard to expel the faecal matter. Never ignore the urge to pass a bowel movement.

Loose watery faeces—diarrhoea

Sometimes we will have bouts of these types of bowel movements when we have a viral or bacterial infection. If you are experiencing this type constantly, please visit your doctor and get it checked out. Watery bowel movements may leave you very dehydrated. Some possible causes of a loose bowel movement are: food poisoning, medications like antibiotics or antacids, changes in diet, spicy foods, herbal supplements, stress or anxiety, infection, food intolerances, or Irritable Bowel Syndrome (IBS).

Mucous in faeces

You may notice that there is an excessive amount of mucous in your faeces. This can be caused by many things including food allergies and intolerances, parasites, irritation in the bowel, and ulcerative colitis. It may also indicate that you are eating a diet high in mucous-forming foods like dairy, white flour, white sugar, or one high in red meat.

Blood in the faeces

If you notice blood in your faeces you should get this checked by your doctor immediately. Blood in the faeces may be red, which means it is coming from lower in the bowel, or black, which means it has been partially digested and is coming from higher in the digestive tract. There may be many causes for this, but it is wise to get it checked as soon as possible.

Alternating between loose stools and constipation

Some of the possible causes for this alternation can be IBS, which is aggravated by many foods and other factors, or it may be the result of chronic constipation. IBS will usually have associated symptoms of pain, discomfort, and bloating, together with the alternation of constipation and diarrhoea. There can be other reasons for an alternation between the two types of bowel movements, including spicy foods and not drinking enough water. If you have pain, or are concerned about this, please ensure that you visit your doctor for a correct diagnosis.

Thin faeces

This could mean that the colon has narrowed. There can be many causes of this and, again, it is wise to get this checked out by your doctor.

Food particles in faeces

You may notice food particles in your faeces. This could be a sign that you are not chewing your food very well. A healthy bowel movement should have no undigested food matter in it, apart from flaxseeds, or the outer shells of sweet corn, or something similar. It may also signal that your body is not digesting and breaking down your food properly. If you notice undigested food particles in your faeces quite often, please get it checked by your physician.

Colour in the faeces

There may be times when the colour of your bowel movements

change. This can signal some of the following things:

Green faeces—This can indicate many causes including fast transit though the digestive tract, infectious diarrhoea, food poisoning, bacterial overgrowth, malabsorption, ulcerative colitis, celiac disease, Crohn's disease, or cancer. It can also be caused by some medications like antibiotics, certain laxatives, and some supplements, especially iron, which may also make the stool appear black. I recommend that you visit your doctor and get this checked out if you have this symptom.

Pale brown/cream/white faeces—This could indicate that not enough bile is being excreted by the gallbladder. This could also signify that not enough bile is being manufactured by the liver, or that there is a problem associated with the two organs. This symptom needs to be checked by your doctor as soon as possible.

If you are experiencing abnormal bowel movements, please visit your doctor, naturopath, or natural health professional and get it checked out. Not all causes of abnormal bowel movements are serious, but they can be caused by serious conditions. I know that it can be embarrassing talking about your bowel health, but it is a very important subject and one that your health professional knows a lot about. They will be happy to discuss any problems you are having. I urge you not to ignore your bowel problems; they will have a big impact on your skin condition and overall health. Without addressing your bowel health, your skin may not improve.

Constipation

I do not advocate the use of laxatives; they can become habit forming and do not promote or encourage a bowel to work properly and naturally. An increase of soluble and non-soluble fibre will encourage regularity and more normal bowel movements.

Many, many people are constipated. I believe it is because many now eat a lot of processed food, most of which has little or no fibre left in it. Processed white flour, as well as white rice, has had almost all the fibre removed during processing. Protein foods like meat, cheese, and cottage cheese, to name a few, do not contain any fibre, nor do sugar and alcoholic beverages.

There are two kinds of fibre, soluble and insoluble, and both are beneficial for the body and digestive system. Insoluble fibre soaks up water and adds volume to bowel movements; it does not dissolve and may help to clear out old faecal matter from the bowel wall. Soluble fibre dissolves in water and can be partially digested. Studies suggest this type of fibre can also be beneficial in reducing cholesterol.

To put fibre into context, the average adult needs 30–50 grams of fibre per day to help maintain a healthy digestive tract.

The following abbreviated list of common foods shows their fibre levels. The full listings can be found on the USDA's Food and Nutrition Information Center website.[4]

Description	**Weight (g)**	**Fibre Content per Measure**
Fast food cheeseburger, regular, double patty and bun; plain	160g	1.6
Fast food cheeseburger; single, regular patty; plain	102g	1.0
Fast food English muffin with egg, cheese, and Canadian bacon	137g	0.5
Fast food sundae, hot fudge	158g	0.0
Fast food, pizza chain, 14" pizza, pepperoni topping, regular crust	106g	1.6
Milk shakes, thick chocolate	300g (10.6 fl. oz.)	0.9

4 USDA Food and Nutritional Information Center, https://www.ars.usda.gov/SP2UserFiles/Place/12354500/Data/SR25/nutrlist/sr25w291.pdf

Pie, cherry, commercially prepared	117g (1 piece)	0.9
Rice, white, long-grain, regular, cooked	158g (1 cup)	0.6
Wheat flour, white, all-purpose, enriched, bleached	125g (1 cup)	3.4
Bread, white, commercially prepared (includes soft bread crumbs)	15g (1 slice)	0.6
Cake, angel food, commercially prepared	28g (1 piece)	0.4
Carbonated beverage, cola, contains caffeine	370g (12 fl. oz.)	0.0
Cereals ready-to-eat, Kellogg's Froot Loops	30g (1 cup)	0.6
Cereals ready-to-eat, Kellogg's Frosted Flakes	31g (3/4 cup)	0.6
Cereals ready-to-eat, Kellogg's Corn Flakes	28g (1 cup)	0.7

Here are some more foods and their fibre contents; this time they are whole foods.

Description	Weight (g)	Fibre Content per Measure
Nuts, coconut meat, dried (desiccated), sweetened, shredded	93g (1 cup)	4.2
Nuts, almonds	28.35g (1 oz., 24 nuts)	3.5
Oranges, raw, all commercial varieties	131g (1 orange)	3.1
Raspberries, frozen, red, sweetened	250g (1 cup)	11.0
Papayas, raw	304g (1 papaya)	5.5

Rice, brown, long-grain, cooked	195g (1 cup)	3.5
Soybeans, mature cooked, boiled, without salt	172g (1 cup)	10.3
Rice, white, long-grain, regular, cooked	158g (1 cup)	0.6
Wheat flour, white, all-purpose, enriched, bleached	125g (1 cup)	3.4
Wheat flour, whole grain	120g (1 cup)	14.6
Barley, pearled, cooked	157g (1 cup)	6.0
Beans, baked, canned, plain or vegetarian	254g (1 cup)	10.4
Beans, navy, mature seeds, cooked, boiled, without salt	182g (1 cup)	19.1
Bread, whole wheat, commercially prepared	28g (1 slice)	1.9
Cereals ready-to-eat, Quaker 100% Natural Cereal with oats, honey and raisins	51g (1/2 cup)	3.3
Cereals, oats, regular and quick and instant, unenriched, cooked with water (includes boiling and microwaving), without salt	234g (1 cup)	4.0

You can see the difference between whole foods and commercially produced and processed foods. To increase your fibre intake, ensure you eat whole foods; by this I mean foods in their whole state that are unprocessed. Trade white bread for whole wheat bread. Eat fruits with their skin on. Snack on fibre-rich foods like apples and nuts. For breakfast, choose whole grain cereals instead of processed ones. Add beans, lentils, fruits, and vegetables to your diet, and ensure that these items make up the bulk of your food intake.

It is very important to get adequate amounts of fibre in your diet.

There are fibre supplements available; ensure you drink plenty of water with these to avoid further constipation.

There are other causes or contributing factors in constipation like:

- ignoring the urge to defecate
- excessive fibre without adequate water
- stress and/or anxiety
- lack of exercise
- iron supplements
- some medicines and pain killers
- slow transit time due to a lazy bowel or overuse of products like laxatives.

If your bowel has a slow transit time, water will be reabsorbed from the faecal matter, leaving a bowel movement which is hard and difficult to move. If you want to check your transit time, eat a large helping of sweet corn with dinner. You should see the evidence of this corn in your bowel movement before lunchtime the next day. If it takes longer than this to come through, you need to speed up the transit time by increasing your intake of insoluble fibre.

Some of the symptoms of constipation are:

- bad breath
- headaches
- weight gain
- indigestion
- fatigue
- abdominal pain
- bloating
- feeling of being full
- inability to expel a bowel movement, but feeling like you need to
- after having a bowel movement you still feel full
- not having a bowel movement every day
- faeces come out in small, hard pellets.

These are just some symptoms; however, constipation symptoms are wide and varied so you may experience others. Constipation and straining to have a bowel movement may cause other problems like haemorrhoids (piles). As I have already said, I promote addressing constipation without constantly using laxatives. Chronic, long-term constipation can be cured by making dietary and lifestyle changes. These beneficial changes should be permanent, to ensure continued good bowel health.

Chapter 9

Bowel Bacteria

Our bowel houses a large amount of bacteria, some of it beneficial and some of it not. In fact, it can contain over five hundred different types of beneficial bacteria. When the bowel contains adequate amounts of beneficial bacteria, it works properly, digests foods well, and absorbs nutrients properly. In fact, the beneficial bacteria actually play a part in the synthesis of B-group vitamins. Having a high proportion of good bacteria will also help inhibit bad bacteria growth. In addition to helping the digestive system function correctly, beneficial bacteria stimulate and support the immune system. Without an adequate supply of beneficial bacteria, food moves slowly through the bowel, fermenting and rotting as it goes along, creating more toxins and problems for the body.

Some of the initial stores of beneficial bacteria come from our mothers, and we are born with a small supply of them. Breast milk (especially colostrum) provides many different strains of beneficial bacteria. It is becoming more and more common for babies to be formula fed and they are missing out on that initial dose of vital bacteria needed for good digestion. Some companies are now including beneficial bacteria in their baby formula, as the importance of the correct amount in the gut is being recognised.

Some other things that affect good bacteria are antibiotics, stress, preservatives, alcohol, medications (especially antibiotics and oral contraceptive tablets), and certain kinds of foods, especially sugar, as this promotes the growth of bad bacteria and destroys some of the good. Other elements which can affect good bacteria are overeating, coffee, and tobacco. Overeating can actually *destroy* beneficial bacteria. Chlorinated water not only kills bacteria in the water that can make us sick, but may also kill beneficial bacteria in your digestive tract.

Some signs of a bacteria imbalance are, but not limited to:

- bloating
- bad breath
- food allergies/intolerances
- skin conditions
- constipation
- diarrhoea
- digestive disturbances
- gas
- heartburn
- body odour
- candida
- hay fever
- sugar cravings

Luckily, it is very easy to re-inoculate the bowel with good bacteria. Probiotics are readily available and contain billions of beneficial bacteria in every capsule. You can use natural yoghurt, as it contains all or some of the following beneficial bacteria: lactobacillus acidophilus, lactobacillus bulgaricus, or lactobacillus casei. It will take significant amounts of yoghurt to get enough good bacteria to restore the bowel, especially if your stores are very low.

Most commercially produced yoghurts are sweetened and this may destroy some of the beneficial bacteria. Also, digestion will kill a lot of the bacteria before it gets into the lower bowel where it is needed. It is estimated that even when probiotic capsules are in a safety coating, only 30–65 percent of the bacteria survive the journey through the digestive tract. I believe that probiotics are your best choice when trying to re-inoculate the bowel with good bacteria; they are convenient, readily available, and easy to take.

Who should take probiotics? Every person who has ever been on antibiotics; you should re-inoculate the bowel with good bacteria every time you take antibiotics. You should regularly take probiotics if you take an oral contraceptive pill or painkillers. You should take a course of probiotics if you have had a stressful event in your life, if you drink alcohol, or eat a diet high in sugar and white flour.

In fact, I recommend that everyone take a course of good-quality probiotics at least once a year, more often if you have any symptoms that show an imbalance may be present.

Chapter 10

Food Allergies/Intolerances

Food allergies and intolerances could be contributing to your skin condition. Food allergies can give the following symptoms: joint pain, migraines, headaches, asthma, eczema, skin conditions, cravings, itchy skin, rapid heartbeat, irritability, dizziness, exhaustion, and insomnia, to name just a few. The following instant allergy check is extracted, with permission, from *Hidden Food Allergies*[5] by Patrick Holford and Dr. James Braly, a book I highly recommend. To see if food allergies or intolerances may be contributing to your skin condition and your overall digestion, take this quick test.

Your Instant Allergy Check

- Are you chronically tired?
- Can you gain weight in hours?
- Do you get bloated after eating?
- Do you suffer from diarrhoea or constipation?
- Do you suffer from abdominal pain?
- Do you sometimes get sleepy after eating?
- Do you suffer from nasal congestion, sneezing, running nose, etc.?

[5] Dr. James Braly and Patrick Holford, Hidden Food Allergies (London: Piatkus Books, Ltd., 2005)

- Do you suffer from rashes, itches, asthma, or shortness of breath?
- Do you have recurrent colds or sinus problems?
- Do you suffer from water retention?
- Do you suffer from migraines or headaches?
- Do you suffer from other aches or pains from time to time, possibly after certain foods?
- Do you suffer from "brain fog" or patches of inexplicable depression?
- Do you get better on holidays abroad, when your diet is completely different?

If you answered yes to any of these questions, it means there is a real possibility that you have an allergy. If you score four or more yeses, it's pretty much guaranteed.

There are two types of food allergies, immediate onset, and delayed onset.

There are laboratory tests which can be done to assess food allergies and intolerances; this involves pricking the skin and putting a test product on it, looking for reactions. These skin tests only tend to show immediate onset allergies. There are other tests that can be done in a laboratory; however, these still often don't expose all allergies.

Only about 5 percent of those affected have immediate-onset food allergies (IgE) and this type is pretty obvious. Immediately after eating the allergenic food you may have physical symptoms like rashes, hives, and itching, or more severe symptoms like swelling of the lips, tongue, or throat. More severely, you can experience anaphylaxis, which is a whole-body reaction to an agent and is life threatening unless treated immediately.

The classic symptoms are well documented in *In Hidden Food Allergies*:

The skin, gut, and airways are the usual arena for IgE allergic reactions. So you may see a rash, urticaria (nettle rash) or eczema. You may start to vomit, or experience nausea, stomach cramps, dull aching, bloating, heartburn, indigestion, constipation, flatulence or diarrhoea. (Most people diagnosed with irritable bowel syndrome are found to have food allergies). Other immediate symptoms include the coughing and wheezing associated with asthma or the sneezing and stuffy nose of a person with allergic rhinitis. The frequency and severity of the reactions vary greatly from person to person.

At the extreme end of the scale. The person can develop anaphylaxis—a reaction where throat and mouth swell and severe asthma comes on, resulting in death from suffocation.

Anaphylactic reactions can also include a kind of nettle rash, rapid dropping of blood pressure, an irregular heartbeat, and loss of consciousness.

Here are some of the more common conditions where IgE food allergy may play a part:

- Allergic dermatitis, eczema
- Angioedema (swelling of the skin, for example on the lips)
- Psoriasis
- Asthma
- Interstitial cystitis (recurrent urinary infections with no known cause)
- Epilepsy
- Non-seasonal allergic rhinitis (nasal irritation not connected to hay fever, for instance)
- Ulcerative colitis
- Crohn's disease

Delayed onset food allergies are much more common that the IgE type in both children and adults, affecting as many as one in three people—and among those with chronic conditions unresponsive to conventional medicine, up to 70%.

Also known as type-3 allergies, these occur when your immune system creates an overabundance of IgG antibodies to a particular food allergen. The antibodies, instead of attaching to mast cells like their IgE counterparts, bind directly to the food particles as they enter your bloodstream, creating immune complexes. The more of these you have floating around the bloodstream, the more on edge your immune system becomes, sending out phagocytes to gobble the complexes up. Basically, your immune system gradually goes into red alert.

This process takes time, which is why IgG symptoms are delayed and only appear two hours to several days after consuming the allergen. For examples, a migraine headache characteristically appears 48 hours after the allergen is eaten.

These delayed reactions can involve almost any organ or tissue in the human body, potentially provoking over 100 allergic symptoms and implicated in well over 100 medical diseases and conditions. Here is a partial list of the more common conditions caused or aggravated by IgG food allergy.

- Allergic rhinitis, non-seasonal
- Anxiety, panic attacks
- Asthma (may involve both IgG and IgE antibodies at the same time)
- Attention deficit hyperactivity disorder (ADHD)
- Autism (associated with milk and gluten cereal allergies)

- Bed wetting
- Depression
- Diabetes, insulin-dependent (gluten, soya and milk casein are primary culprits)
- Eczema (may involve both IgG and IgE antibodies at the same time)
- Epilepsy (with history of migraines or hyperactivity)
- Fatigue, chronic
- Fibromyalgia
- Headaches (migraines, cluster)
- Inflammatory bowel disease (cow's milk enterocolitis, Crohn's disease, ulcerative colitis, and celiac disease\ iron deficient anaemia
- Irritable bowel syndrome
- Middle ear disease (acute or serious otitis media)
- Rheumatoid arthritis
- Sleep disorders (insomnia, sleep apnoea, snoring)

Any estimated one in four people suffer from clinically significant food allergies, most of them from delayed symptoms that are probably the result of IgG food allergies. Unlike IgE allergies, IgG food allergies are very common and rarely self-diagnosed or treated.

Immediate food allergy can often be diagnosed with a simple skin test. Delayed reactions to food often require state of the art blood tests that detect the presence of specific IgG antibodies to foods in your blood.

It may be quite complex to find out what foods you are allergic or intolerant to. Then, of course, there is a lot of debate over which tests work and which don't. Doctors favour skin testing and RAST blood testing, but this will only diagnose an IgE food allergy. They do not expose an IgG food allergy—the most common type. There are now IgG ELISA home tests available. This involves a small finger prick, extracting some blood onto an absorbent material, and sending it to a lab for testing. Depending on the lab processing the sample, it is usual for about a hundred foods to be tested. You get a printout returned showing foods which must be completely avoided, and those which just need to be rotated and can be eaten every four days or so. You can find many different companies providing these tests online. There is controversy about this test—but isn't there always!

There are two other tests I favour. You can test yourself using the pulse-testing system. Take your pulse rate over a minute. Do this several times a day, so you will get to know your average pulse. Now, after you eat a meal take your pulse at intervals of fifteen, thirty, and forty-five minutes. If you have an allergy to a food that you have consumed, your pulse rate will rise by at least ten beats per minute. This is because an allergy to a food will cause the release of adrenalin, which will increase your heart rate. This is an easy test and can help you begin to define any possible food allergies.

If you have had a meal consisting of egg and bread and find an increase in the pulse rate, you will need to define whether it is the egg or the bread (perhaps the wheat or gluten), so you will need to repeat the test after just eating an egg, and then another day after just eating bread. The upside of this test is that it is free! But it can be quite time consuming.

Another way to find out any food intolerances is by getting an EAV test. Using a hair sample, a test is done to assess what foods you are allergic or intolerant to. You are then provided with a written report showing which foods you need to steer clear of.

If you are intolerant or allergic to some foods, take heart in knowing if you remove that food from your diet, and use a probiotic which will fill the bowel with beneficial bacteria and help the bowel wall to heal or repair, you may be able to reintroduce this food at a later stage and have no reaction. I would recommend removing any intolerant food from your diet for at least six months before trying it again. This means removing the food completely, not consuming it at all. You cannot simply reduce the reactive food and expect to repair the intolerant or allergic reaction. You must completely remove it. This entails reading labels and ensuring that you are not unwittingly eating even small portions of the offending food.

One easy way to help ensure that you are not reacting to food allergies or intolerances is to vary your diet day to day and meal to meal. If you have toast for breakfast, have no other wheat products during that day. For lunch, have a mixed salad with some tuna. For dinner, have a baked potato and steamed vegetables. Have two snacks during the day.

The most common foods that people with skin conditions are allergic or intolerant to are wheat, citrus fruits, and dairy.

Take notice of how you feel, begin to write a diary of how you feel each day, and then notice if there are any patterns. Food intolerances/allergies may make you tired or your heart may race. Write down any physical symptoms and look for recurring patterns. Perhaps you feel really, really tired and you begin to notice that this is the case after you have eaten a lot of bread. This will be a sign of intolerance to bread—perhaps the wheat, yeast, or gluten. Any one of these may be the component that causes the problem, or perhaps you are intolerant to them all. If you are having reactions from bread, my advice is to completely remove it, regardless of whether you know which ingredient in it you are allergic to.

Today, there is a large number of people who are now intolerant to wheat and other products. Food producers are becoming more aware of this and every year there are more and more alternatives to wheat products available. Don't be afraid that you'll have nothing left to eat if you remove all the foods you suspect you are intolerant to.

Chapter 11

Liver Dysfunction

Your body cannot digest food properly if your liver is not functioning well.

The liver has many jobs. In fact it is one of the most important organs in the body, due to its many functions. It synthesises protein; synthesises, stores, and processes fats, fatty acids, and cholesterol; metabolises and stores carbohydrates; makes and secretes bile, which aids in digestion; eliminates harmful compounds from the blood (including alcohol and medicine); and detoxifies the body by breaking down or changing chemicals, waste, and toxins so that they can be excreted.

If your liver is not functioning properly you may have symptoms including (but not limited to):

- excessive cholesterol and fats in arteries
- weight gain
- inability to lose weight even when dieting
- fatty build up in organs
- lumps of fat appearing in skin
- gall bladder stones
- slow metabolism
- intolerance to fat or alcohol
- sugar cravings
- nausea and vomiting

- constipation
- IBS (irritable bowel syndrome)
- depression
- poor concentration
- brain fog
- headaches
- skin rashes
- chronic fatigue syndrome
- bad breath
- excessive sweating
- dark circles under the eyes
- yellow discolouration in the eyes
- body odour
- hormone imbalance
- PMS
- allergies like hives, hay fever, dermatitis, asthma and sinusitis
- digestive problems
- stomach pains
- feeling of fullness after meals

This is not a complete list and these symptoms may be caused by other factors, but if you are suffering from any of these it could be an indication that your liver is not functioning correctly.

If you have some of these symptoms, and suspect you have liver dysfunction, please visit your doctor to get checked, as liver disease needs to be diagnosed and treated early. A simple blood sample will help expose any major dysfunction or disease. However, Dr. Sandra Cabot, who wrote the famous book *The Liver Cleansing Diet*, says it is possible for people to have a dysfunctional liver, even though the blood tests show normal results. Sometimes, even a small reduction in liver function can cause a lot of symptoms in the body.

You can, however, begin to support your liver and therefore increase its function. The easiest way this can be done is with dietary changes. Our diet may be the biggest contributing factor to liver dysfunction.

What to eat to support the liver

The liver is an amazing organ and has an incredible capacity to repair itself, if given the support needed. Many herbs and foods will support and enable the liver to detoxify and regenerate. By assisting the liver function better you will have increased overall good health. Eating a balanced diet with limited artificial ingredients is the simplest way to support and help repair this important organ. By providing it with adequate nutrients your whole body will be able to repair itself and function properly.

Eat lots of fresh raw vegetables, sprouts, and fresh fruits. Mix the colours of the fruits and vegetables, because the different colours contain different vitamins, minerals, and antioxidants. Lightly steam vegetables that you prefer cooked. Eat brown rice and other whole grains. As often as possible, buy organic to reduce the amount of sprays and chemicals that you are ingesting from your food. Also, drink adequate amounts of water to ensure you aid in the elimination of toxins.

What to remove from your diet to support your liver

You should avoid alcohol, preservatives, artificial colours and additives, and sugar. Processed foods often have many of the nutrients removed. Steer clear of white flour products like cakes, white bread, white rice, and pasta. If you cannot live without these foods, eat them in moderation occasionally, but substitute them with whole grain varieties when you do.

Read the labels on what you are eating. Take charge of your health and what you put into your body. Change to brands that have no added preservatives or chemical additives. Foods high in saturated fats should be limited or avoided because they make the liver work harder during the digestion process. Limit, or avoid completely, caffeinated drinks including coffee, energy drinks, and sodas. Have these as treats, not as daily drinks.

Ready-to-eat supermarket meals and fast foods often have preservatives and artificial ingredients added to them to aid in the manufacturing process. Read the labels.

Chapter 12

Water

I believe that another significant problem is that people do not drink enough water and are constantly dehydrated. Often, the only fluid intake some people have is in the form of sugary, caffeinated drinks. Dehydration causes a huge number of symptoms and some real problems for the body, especially when it comes to eliminating waste.

Some symptoms of dehydration are (but not limited to):

- headaches
- decreased urination
- dry skin
- dry lips
- thirst
- fatigue and nausea
- dry mouth
- fatigue or weakness
- head rushes
- chills

If dehydration continues, the symptoms will worsen and become more serious, and may include some of the following symptoms:

- increased heart rate
- increased respiration

- decreased sweating
- decreased urination
- increased body temperature
- extreme fatigue
- muscle cramps
- headaches
- nausea
- tingling of the limbs
- loss of consciousness

You can easily tell if you are dehydrated. One way is that your urine will appear dark yellow. When you are well hydrated, your urine will be straw coloured or almost clear. Often, we wait until we are thirsty before we have a drink, but by the time you're thirsty you will already be dehydrated. If your lips are dry, then you are dehydrated. Also, the older you get, the slower the signal mechanisms work. So, if you are over fifty and feel thirsty, then you will already be significantly dehydrated.

Another factor in dehydration is that we often eat when we are actually thirsty, mistaking the signals our bodies are giving us; and that keeps us constantly dehydrated. I also think you should be drinking pure water, not these new supplement waters or flavoured waters. Often, these flavoured waters contain artificial sweeteners, flavours, preservatives, sugar, and vitamins that are not beneficial for our bodies. You are just adding another component to your diet that your body has to dispose of which may prolong your condition. All you need is pure, fresh water with nothing added.

During your treatment your body is detoxifying and eliminating waste, so you need to ensure that you drink two litres of water per day. I know that this can be challenging for some people. I suggest carrying around a sipper bottle everywhere you go. This way you'll be able to monitor your water consumption. Also, you can slowly sip away all day and, after a few days, you will need to go to the bathroom less as your body adjusts to the higher fluid intake. The membranes in your mouth can absorb water, so sipping slowly aids this, rather than drinking large quantities at once. Drinking too much water at once will overwhelm your system and will often seem to go straight through you.

Section 4

The Treatment

Chapter 13

Supplements I Used to Cure My Psoriasis and Other Symptoms

Apart from the skin lesions, I had constipation. I did not drink enough water, and I had some digestive complaints, like feeling bloated after a meal, and feeling full for hours. This chapter contains information about the supplements I used to treat my psoriasis. In later chapters, I will give you information to help you decide what supplements you may need to add to your regime.

Supplements I used

Red clover combination capsules

I used a red clover combination with prickly ash bark. The formula I used contained red clover, prickly ash bark, buckthorn, sarsaparilla, burdock, liquorice, barberry, echinacea purpurea, cascara sagrada, sheep sorrel, and rosemary. Do *not* use plain red clover capsules; find a combination capsule containing similar ingredients to this.

The formula I used cleanses the blood and lymphatic system. It also cleanses the bowel and has laxative qualities to promote evacuation. It removes accumulated toxins and waste. It has anti-parasitic, antiseptic qualities, and it stimulates the immune system. Digestion can be improved and the liver may be stimulated to produce more bile. The ingredients are known to cleanse the liver, bowel, blood, and lymphatic system. It will help open up elimination channels, and is a diuretic to decrease fluid retention. These ingredients are also known for their traditional use in treating psoriasis.

Precautions

Do not take if pregnant or breastfeeding. Before taking any supplements check with your doctor or natural health professional, especially if you are taking other medications. Do not use if you have diarrhoea or abdominal pains. Reduce dosage, or discontinue use, if abdominal pain or diarrhoea develops.

The initial dosage I used was one capsule, three times a day. Every week I increased the dose by one capsule per day until I was taking three capsules, three times a day. Although this differs from the directions on the label, it was the manufacturer's suggested dosage that I received as a practitioner. When you buy your red clover formula, talk to your natural health care professional at your health food shop, and get them to check the manufacturer-suggested maximum dosage.

Keep taking this formula, even after your lesions have begun to get better. This is very important, because if you stop taking the red clover combination prematurely, your lesions will get worse. Once all your lesions are healed, it may be necessary to stay on it to stop them from coming back. I recommend staying on a dose of one tablet daily, and increasing it if the lesions start to come back.

Digestive enzymes

Because I suspected that I also did not produce enough digestive enzymes, I also took an enzyme supplement with every meal. Some signs of an enzyme deficiency are (but not limited to):

- acne
- bladder problems
- psoriasis
- constipation
- diarrhoea
- chronic allergies

- irritable bowel
- indigestion and gas

Digestive enzymes are necessary for the correct digestion of your food. They help to break down food particles, and they help your body to assimilate the nutrients from food. Our modern diets are often also full of cooked, processed, and fast foods. The enzymes in these types of foods have been killed during the manufacturing or cooking process, and have virtually no live enzymes left in them. If your diet is low in live, unprocessed raw foods, then you will probably be lacking in digestive enzymes and you may need supplements as I did. We also produce fewer enzymes as we age.

Food that is not digested properly becomes fuel for bad bacteria. It can also begin to ferment in the bowel, creating even more toxins and problems. Digestion is a very important function affecting every body system, and it is important to ensure that you are digesting food correctly.

Probiotics

Probiotics are a supplement that contains millions of live beneficial bacteria. The bowel needs certain types of beneficial bacteria to digest food properly, and to assimilate adequate nutrients from our food. The bowel holds a huge amount of bacteria, both beneficial and harmful. A diet high in sugar, alcohol, and processed foods will encourage the growth of bad bacteria and may inhibit the growth of the good. This causes an imbalance which may manifest itself in many like (but not limited to):

- tiredness
- bloating
- gas
- constipation
- diarrhoea
- heartburn

- food sensitivities
- cravings for carbohydrates and/or sugar
- headaches
- nausea

Some medications, like the contraceptive pill and antibiotics, also kill good bacteria. It is imperative that you have adequate amounts of good bacteria in your bowel to ensure good bowel health and effective digestion.

I took several courses of probiotics. Even though I have not been prescribed many courses of antibiotics during my lifetime, my diet (which earlier on in my life wasn't very good) meant that my large intestine was probably full of non-beneficial bacteria. I had also taken oral contraceptives for many years. I had symptoms of my bacteria being out of balance—constipation, discomfort, and digestive problems. All this led me to believe that it would be wise to re-inoculate my bowel with beneficial bacteria.

Multi-vitamins

I used a good-quality organic spirulina. This was my choice to enhance my nutrient intake. I like taking supplements that I feel that my body can assimilate quite easily. For me, this means choosing a plant-based natural supplement, as some companies add minerals to their supplements that have been mined out of the ground and our bodies are simply unable to assimilate them. So, while you think you are doing something good for your body, you can actually be creating more problems. Price is always a sign of a good-quality product. I do not buy the cheap supplements, because often they are produced without as much research as the higher priced ones, and they are made with lower-quality ingredients.

Spirulina contains eight essential amino acids, ten non-essential amino acids, minerals, and vitamins. It also contains precursors necessary for your body to synthesize vitamins. As well as all this, it has other active ingredients and provides protein. It is also said to help build and enrich the blood, enhance intestinal flora, detoxify the kidneys and liver, and nourish the body.

I also use other multi-vitamin supplements when I feel I need a boost. I personally choose supplements that are made with plant-based materials. I do not recommend staying permanently on any multi-vitamin or mineral supplement. Supplements are not a substitute for cleaning up your diet; they are an interim product which can help your body restore its nutrient balance. Your main intake of nutrients should always come from your food.

Fibre

I increased the amount of fibre in my diet, and I took supplement capsules to make sure I was taking in an adequate amount to keep my bowel working properly, and to ensure that all toxins and old faecal matter were being removed.

As you have seen in previous chapters, there is a large difference in the fibre levels between whole grains and refined products. By choosing whole grains, you will be increasing the fibre level considerably. Not only do whole grain foods contain more fibre, they also usually contain more nutrients.

Essential omega-3 oils

There is a lot of evidence that suggests omega oils are effective in helping treat skin conditions. Omega-3 oils have been shown to be quite effective in the study referenced below. Whilst you can obtain omega-3 from fish oils, it can also be obtained from other food sources including flaxseeds, walnuts, soybeans, navy beans, kidney beans, grape seed oil, and tofu.

The following abstract came from *PubMed*[6]:

6 "A double-blind, randomised, placebo-controlled trial of fish oil in psoriasis," PubMed.gov website, http://www.ncbi.nlm.nih.gov/pubmed/2893189?

A double-blind, randomised, placebo-controlled trial of fish oil in psoriasis.

The Lancet, February 20, 1988, pp. 378–80

By Bittiner SB, Tucker WF, Cartwright I, Bleehen SS

Department of Dermatology, Royal Hallamshire Hospital, Sheffield.

28 patients with stable chronic psoriasis completed a trial in which they were randomly allocated to receive either 10 fish-oil capsules ('MaxEPA') or 10 placebo capsules (olive oil) daily. Patients were specifically instructed not to change their normal diet. After 8 weeks' treatment there was a significant lessening of itching, erythema*, and scaling in the active treatment group, with a trend towards an overall decrease in body surface area affected. No change occurred in the placebo group.

(*erythema is the redness of the skin caused by dilatation and congestion of the capillaries, often a sign of inflammation or infection.)

It really comes down to your personal preference. Some people can easily add omega-rich foods into their diet, while others struggle and require supplementation. I suggest that you take omega oils for a few months or whilst your skin is healing. If you do not have many omega-3-rich foods in your diet, then it may be necessary to continue to take a supplement. Talk to a natural health professional at your shop for further advice and help with choosing an appropriate form of omega oil for you.

Chapter 14

Dietary Alterations

I had to make some dietary alterations. I had to be realistic and accept that my diet played a huge part in my skin condition. My psoriasis wasn't a punishment from God, and I wasn't just unlucky. My condition had definite causes and contributing factors, and my diet was a major contributor. This was probably the most difficult aspect of my healing. Changing your diet is never easy, especially when you've had a habit of eating a certain way for a long time. Please don't skip making dietary changes as they will not only help the healing of your skin, they will also help in the overall improvement of your health and wellbeing.

Water

I increased the amount of water I drank to help my body deal with the toxins that were being flushed from my body, and it also helped with my constipation. I drank two litres per day of filtered water. It is not necessary to buy spring water; invest in a good-quality filter and refill bottles at home.

Decrease sugar

I decreased the amount of sugar that I was having in a day. I believe sugar can be quite destructive to the body. I swapped sugary cups of coffee for water, or I swapped the sugar for stevia. Stevia is a herb which is virtually calorie free and is many times sweeter than sugar. It can be used to sweeten beverages and used in baking as a sugar alternative. Just a few drops in a cup of coffee will sweeten it.

I do not recommend the use of artificial sweeteners. I believe that the fewer artificial ingredients and chemicals you put into the body the better.

Diet changes

I began to take notice of how I felt after meals. If I ate a meal and it felt like a lump in my stomach afterwards, then I would avoid this food, especially certain types of meat. Pork generally makes me feel unwell. I have since read recommendations that all people with psoriasis should refrain completely from eating pork, and pork products, like bacon, ham, bologna, and sausages.

I reduced the amount of bad fat in my diet and began to use olive oil and other beneficial oils for cooking. I also cut the fat off meats before I cooked them to remove the temptation to eat it.

I reduced the amount of artificial ingredients and preservatives that I was eating. I stopped buying foods that were pre-prepared, and began to make more of my own. Meatloaf is filled with fat and artificial ingredients when you buy it prepared, but it is easy to make out of lean meat and it tastes great. I began to take notice of packaging and ingredients, and stopped buying foods that had artificial sweeteners, additives, and preservatives. You will be absolutely blown away by the foods that are full of preservatives—salamis, bacon, sliced meats, ham, and sausages. In fact, anything that can sit in your refrigerator for an extended period will probably have preservatives in it. Look at your canned goods, like baked beans or spaghetti, and swap to another brand that does not contain preservatives. Check your pasta sauces and other bottled foods for the use of preservatives, as there are many brands available without them.

Instead of using preservative-rich foods in salads like ham, I used tuna in spring water, salmon, or leftover chicken or turkey from dinner.

I know that this sounds like a lot of work, but I just learned to make exchanges for healthier options. I would exchange white bread for whole grain bread, and I would exchange a sweet biscuit for a rice cracker and cheese. I ate more whole grains and had things like porridge or fruit for breakfast. At lunchtime I had a whole grain bun filled with salads, or a salad by itself. At night I had fish, chicken, lamb, or beef with vegetables, rather than having sausages or processed foods. It took some time to change my eating habits and to adjust to the new foods, and perhaps my diet will always be a work in progress. Some days I still slip into old habits but, fairly quickly, I would begin to feel physically bad and know I have to change back to my healthier choices.

I still allow myself treats, but just keep them limited and don't indulge every day. Sometimes it was difficult to change, but I found that the most important thing was to be organised and ensure I planned my meals and had healthy alternatives available for snacks.

I have added a chapter about dietary considerations, and a sample diet plan, to make this easier for you. It is important that you restrict your intake of harmful foods. By doing this, you will speed up your body's ability to detoxify and begin the healing of your skin, because you will not be taking in more toxins and overloading your system.

Chapter 15

Recommended Diet

I believe that the diet has a huge effect on psoriasis. I recommend dietary changes to all my clients who suffer from it. Some changes are easy to make and others take some effort, but it is important that you do make some changes. Your diet *has* contributed to your skin condition, and if you do not make changes you will never escape your psoriasis prison. Hopefully, I have given you enough information so that you can now understand the correlation between digestion and the overall health of your body.

Although you may now understand the importance of having a healthy diet, do not make all the changes in one week. Make them slowly so it will be easier to follow and stick to. You have had your old eating habits for a long time, and it is going to take some time to change them. Your first step can be to remove foods you should no longer eat from your pantry so that they will not entice you to eat them.

Remove from your diet

There are some factors that need to be removed from your diet, at least until your psoriasis subsides.

Allergic/intolerant foods—it is necessary for you to remove any food from your diet that you are allergic or intolerant to. Instructions for pulse testing have been listed earlier in this book; or it's possible to get a test done to assess the foods you should additionally remove from your diet. These may include dairy foods, orange juice, and wheat products. You may notice after eating some foods your lesions become itchy or irritated. Start to take notice of what different foods do to your skin, and write a diary listing and noting any reactions to see if there is a pattern forming. Sometimes the reaction may take up to forty-eight hours to manifest itself, and by writing a diary it will be easy to see any patterns.

Alcohol—I really recommend that you stop drinking alcoholic beverages. I know that there are some antioxidant benefits of certain types of alcohol, but for the sake of a speedy recovery, stop drinking, at least for the time being. Personally, I had stopped drinking alcohol over ten years ago, so this was not an issue for me.

Fizzy drinks—swap sugared, carbonated drinks for plain water. I am not a fan of artificial sweeteners. I would prefer you switched to water rather than artificially sweetened fizzy drinks. Fizzy drinks not only contain sugar that we want to remove from our diet, but also artificial colours, flavours, and additives. Plain, filtered water is a far better option. If you must have fizzy drinks, have them as a treat and don't have them every day.

Fruit juices—if you can't do without your usual fruit juices, water them down. Take a moment to think about a glass of juice. It may take ten or twelve individual pieces of fruit to make a cup of juice. Realistically, you would not eat that many pieces of fruit in a sitting. Sometimes, commercially produced juices contain mould and particles of rotten fruit that have passed through their quality control. You wouldn't juice rotten fruit and drink it. It's about knowing what is in what you eat and drink.

Cakes, white flour sugary bakery goods—often these baked goods contain lots of sugar, and very little fibre and nutrients. Some bakeries use premixed bases or cake mixes, which contain artificial ingredients and sweeteners. They may also use margarine instead of butter. So as you can see, commercially prepared goods can be full of sugar, additives, artificial sweeteners, colourings, and flavourings. If you must have baked goods, try healthier options like those made with whole grains, or wheat, and gluten-free options.

Processed foods and meals—processing methods often use artificial ingredients and modified ingredients which can create problems within the body. Often they contain artificial flavourings, colourings, and preservatives, and have fewer nutrients than their homemade counterparts.

Know what is in your food. When you make things yourself, you know exactly what is in it. If you do buy pre-made foods, look for those with no artificial ingredients or preservatives. If you can't read the ingredients, don't buy it. I know it can be more time consuming to make your meals from scratch, but if you get yourself organised it is not very difficult.

What to add to your diet

Fresh vegetables, sprouts, and fruit should make up a large proportion of your diet. Unsweetened natural yoghurt is allowed. Brown rice is a good alternative to white rice and other carbohydrates.

Eat lean meats, not sausages, boloneys, or meat products containing preservatives and additives. Choose meats that are whole and in their natural state. Organic is best. Keep red meats to a minimum, and eat more oily fish that will provide omega-3 oils to your diet; salmon, tuna, mackerel, sardines, herrings, as well as lean chicken and turkey.

If you are not intolerant to wheat, you may have breads but choose whole grain versions that have more nutrients and fibre. Also, choose ones that have no preservatives and artificial ingredients. Organic is best.

Drink two litres per day—I cannot stress this enough. This will help ensure toxins are removed easier, and your body will work better because it is hydrated. Dehydration may be contributing to your constipation, so ensuring you are adequately hydrated may help your bowel.

Sample seven-day diet

This sample seven-day diet will help you to make some changes and give you some ideas. It is a low-reactive diet, which may be helpful, and I have kept out the most reactive foods like wheat, citrus, and dairy (excluding yoghurt, which is usually tolerated even by those with a dairy intolerance). You can use this as a guide to start with. If you find that you feel unwell, tired, or bloated after a meal, then it may be necessary for you to alter that meal, as one of the foods in it doesn't agree with you.

The easiest way to make the transition to a better diet is to be really organised, and ensure your cupboards are full of the ingredients that you need to make your meals. Fill your vegetable bin with lots of green leafy vegetables and sprouts. Plan the week's meals so you do not get caught and turn to processed or fast foods.

If you wish to make up your own meals, try and make sure your plate consists of at least 50 percent vegetables, and one serving of protein—chicken, fish, beef, lamb, or turkey. You do not have to have a protein component in every meal; include some vegetarian meals. When you have a protein meal, a serving is about a palm-sized piece. One serving of carbohydrate foods, like brown rice, quinoa, and potatoes, is about a handful. The rest of your plate should consist of vegetables.

Be aware of your serving sizes, as often we eat far too much. Initially, put less on your plate and chew your food very well to aid in digestion. Wait a few minutes after you finish your plate before you serve yourself any more. Often, by the time you feel full you have usually already eaten too much. By waiting a while before eating more, you may find that you do not need that second helping. It just takes a few minutes to feel full. Be aware that overeating may exacerbate your psoriasis, because it overloads the digestive system and may prevent the body from digesting your meal properly.

SEVEN-DAY SAMPLE DIET

Day One

Breakfast: Rice porridge: put ½ cup rice milk or water and 1 cup cooked brown rice into a saucepan, bring to the boil, and simmer for 10–20 minutes until it reaches the desired consistency, similar to oatmeal.

Morning snack: Carrot sticks and hummus (chickpea dip—make yourself or buy readymade, but ensure you buy one that does not contain preservatives or artificial ingredients); you can also use celery sticks as an alternative.

Lunch: Grilled tuna steak with mixed salad. Include a variety of coloured salad leaves, tomatoes, and cucumber. Dress with lemon or lime juice—can be poured over the fish as well.

Afternoon snack: Smoothie made with soymilk and a banana, blended till smooth; ice may be added if preferred.

Dinner: Grilled chicken and steamed asparagus, zucchini, and broccoli.

Supper: Water and lemon juice to taste or herbal tea (ensure it is natural with no artificial ingredients or flavourings).

Day Two

Breakfast: Poached eggs with sautéed spinach and mushrooms.

Morning snack: Handful of pumpkin seeds.

Lunch: Salmon (fresh or canned), iceberg lettuce, and herbs like parsley and coriander; add some beetroot and other vegetables that you like.

Afternoon snack: Piece of fresh pineapple.

Dinner: Roast lean lamb with roasted vegetables, parsnip, sweet potatoes, and collard greens.

Supper: Herbal tea.

Day Three

Breakfast: Porridge—oats cooked with water, may be served with

soy milk, rice milk or yoghurt.
Morning snack: 1 pear or apple.
Lunch: Sandwich with rye bread or rice bread (ensure it contains no wheat) filled with salad vegetables of your choice. You may add a small amount of butter.
Afternoon snack: Handful of sunflower seeds or walnuts.
Dinner: Cooked cold turkey with a salad made from snow peas, green beans (blanched), celery, and sprouts and dressed with olive oil, lemon juice, herbs, and garlic.
Supper: Ginger tea, using either a bought ginger tea or by simply using a piece of sliced fresh root ginger and pouring boiling water over it, and letting it steep for a few minutes. This may be sweetened with a small amount of stevia or honey if needed.

Day Four
Breakfast: Smoothie with yoghurt and pineapple or mango—add water to thin if too thick.
Morning snack: Rice crackers and canned tuna garnished with alfalfa sprouts.
Lunch: Vegetable soup made from potatoes, carrots, squash, spinach, garlic, tomatoes, broccoli, and onion, or any other favourite vegetables. Sauté onions in a little olive oil until soft and then add other vegetables. Cover with water, organic chicken or vegetable stock, and simmer till tender. Blend until it reaches the desired consistency. Make a large pot and freeze extra servings in single-serve containers.
Afternoon snack: Celery sticks and hummus (chickpea dip).
Dinner: Grilled or steamed fish with mixed salad on the side and baked potato (potato optional).
Supper: Water and lemon juice to taste.

Day Five
Breakfast: Rice porridge: put ½ cup rice milk or water and 1 cup

cooked brown rice into a saucepan, bring to the boil, and simmer for 10–20 minutes until it reaches the desired consistency. Rice milk is quite sweet and you may not need any further sweetening agents.
Morning snack: Vegetable juice made from beetroot, carrots, and celery—dilute so it's easier on your digestive system.
Lunch: Chicken and vegetable stir-fry. Stir fry chicken strips till cooked, remove, and rest on a plate. Stir fry onion and garlic and add your favourite stir-fry vegetables, and mung bean sprouts. Add a little organic chicken stock to flavour it, and to help steam the vegetables. Add your chicken back in to warm back up.
Afternoon snack: 2 fresh kiwifruit (green or yellow).
Dinner: Baked potato with a small pat of butter or olive oil (I prefer not to use margarine, as most of them contain artificial ingredients, additives or modified ingredients). Fresh sweet corn on the cob, and a fresh salad with greens, avocado, tomato, and your other favourite ingredients.
Supper: Herbal tea of your choice.

Day Six

Breakfast: Porridge—oats cooked with water, maybe served with oat milk or yoghurt.
Morning snack: Rice cakes and banana.
Lunch: Chicken and coleslaw. Steamed or grilled chicken breast served with coleslaw, made from cabbage (red or white), scallion or onion (red or white), carrot (grated), tomato, and fresh ground pepper. Use as a dressing a mixture of vinegar or lemon juice and natural yoghurt. You can also add sweet ingredients like pineapple, raisins, and nuts like hazelnuts if you prefer.
Afternoon snack: Piece of fruit of choice (not citrus) or berries.
Dinner: Salmon or tuna patties; mix a tin of salmon or tuna and add to some mashed potato or sweet potato with finely chopped scallion and herbs, season with salt and pepper. Form into patties and pan fry in a little olive oil. Serve with a salad of your choice.

Fresh salmon can be used instead of canned.

Day Seven

Breakfast: Blueberry and rice milk smoothie—frozen berries can be used, other berries may be added if you prefer.

Morning snack: Piece of fruit of choice (not citrus).

Lunch: Pumpkin soup. Chop 2 large onions and sauté in a little olive oil until almost tender, add 1–5 cloves of garlic (to taste) and sauté a few minutes more, add 1–2 tsp. curry powder (optional) and a pinch of cayenne pepper (optional), add 1 medium pumpkin chopped into cubes. Just cover with water or organic chicken or vegetable stock (check for preservatives or additives). Cook until the pumpkin is tender and then blend until desired consistency is reached. Extra water may be added if it is too thick. Cook a large pot full and freeze into single serve containers for a convenient quick lunch idea.

Afternoon snack: Rice crackers and hummus (chickpea dip—make yourself or buy readymade but ensure you buy one that does not contain preservatives or artificial ingredients).

Dinner: Grilled steak, baked potato with a little butter, and a salad of your choice.

Supper: Herbal tea of your choice.

Tips for changing your diet

Make more than you need for dinner and take leftovers to work for lunch the next day. Soups are especially easy, as they can be cooked in a slow cooker overnight or during the day whilst you are at work. It is easy to make a large batch using a slow cooker and freeze the leftovers in single-serve containers. Take these to work for lunch or heat at home for a quick meal.

Instead of skipping breakfast, make a smoothie with natural unsweetened yoghurt and fruit and drink it on your way to work. Carry a water bottle around and sip at it to help easily increase your water intake. Take snacks to work like hummus and rice crackers, a piece of fruit, dried fruits, nuts, or vegetable sticks, rather than having high-sugar snacks.

Write a shopping list and plan your meals for the week. This makes it easier to cook or create a healthy meal in a short space of time, rather than reverting to fast foods or processed convenience foods. Buying real food can be much cheaper than convenience and fast foods, especially if you buy directly from the growers or at a local farmer's market.

Blueberries can be added to porridge for flavouring and as a change. Keep some in the freezer for an easy smoothie ingredient, or eat them frozen as a snack. Dried fruits can be a great standby snack especially while on the run. Look for fruits dried naturally, rather than ones preserved with chemicals. Organic is always best. Put into snack-sized bags ready to easily grab. Do the same with organic nuts and seeds.

Vary your diet every day; don't get stuck eating the same things day in and day out, as this may begin a pattern of creating a deficiency. It will also ensure you don't get bored and revert to old habits.

Swap margarine, containing preservatives and artificial ingredients, for natural butter which usually contains only cream and salt (find a natural brand). Use in moderation.

Eat many different coloured vegetables and fruits. The different colours contain different antioxidants, vitamins, and minerals. Eat fruits and vegetables that are in season and local. This will save you money and ensure the fruits and vegetables you are eating are fresh and still full of nutrients.

Eat in moderation; don't eat huge amounts of any one thing. Stop eating before you become too full, put less on your plate, and wait a few minutes before getting a second helping, as you may not need it.

Cook the same meals for everyone in the family, rather than you eating a different diet. This will not only make it easier, but maybe everyone in the family will gain improved health.

Do not look at this as a diet, or that you are going without your favourite foods. This is a lifestyle change to regain your physical, skin, and emotional health. It is not a punishment; it is a road to wellness. Praise yourself for making these changes and enjoy the empowerment of taking control of your health and diet.

CHAPTER 16

Lifestyle Changes

A word about stress

Although I didn't notice a worsening of my psoriasis when I was stressed, stress can affect a lot of organs and processes within the body. Stress can affect the brain, liver, adrenals, digestion, blood pressure, and distribution. It can also lead to mineral deficiencies and exhaustion. It can cause depression and anxiety. Stress is not something that should be ignored. It is important for you to find ways to reduce it whenever possible.

In times of stress I use Bach Flower Remedies®. They are fantastic, especially Rescue Remedy®. If you do not have a Bach flower practitioner in your area, go to your local health food shop or pharmacy to see if they stock it. Bach flower remedies are non-addictive, natural remedies made from spring water and flowers (or sometimes crystals, shells, and other things), and preserved, usually with brandy. They are safe for people of all ages. Rescue Remedy is probably the most famous flower remedy, and I feel it is a must for everyone, great for times of stress or trauma. A flower essence practitioner can also mix you a custom-made remedy, specific to any or all of your emotional needs.

This is another great, simple stress remedy. When you feel stressed out, you will notice that you hold your shoulders stiffer, your neck muscles will tighten, and your shoulders will rise up.

Every time you feel yourself getting stressed, get up and stretch your arms above your head, link your hands and stretch, taking a deep breath while you are doing this. Then lower your arms, push your shoulders back down, and take five deep breaths in through your nose and out through your mouth. Just allow yourself to relax.

Meditation can be a great stress reliever. You do not have to sit cross-legged and chant! Take the phone off the hook. Sit comfortably in a chair or lie down, if you prefer. Put on some nice, soft music (not heavy metal or anything too upbeat). Now, just relax and close your eyes. Take notice of your body and begin to consciously relax, starting at your toes and moving up through your body, relaxing all areas. Breathe deeply in through your nose and out through your mouth. Just relax and enjoy the music. It's that easy!

You should take some time to relax every day. You will be surprised what a difference this simple exercise will make in your life. Don't be too concerned about the amount of time you spend meditating, maybe it will suit you to do five minutes today and half an hour tomorrow. As long as you use whatever time you have relaxing, it will be beneficial to you.

Find an activity you enjoy and do it daily to help relieve the stress of daily life. Perhaps you could go for a walk on a beach, or through a forest or park. Maybe you enjoy just sitting quietly admiring your garden or reading a book. Take an approach to do something to relax and enjoy every day.

Exercise

I recommend that if you are not already doing so, that you begin an exercise regime. Exercise is absolutely necessary for overall good health and wellbeing. As you exercise, endorphins will be released that will make you feel good. You will increase your circulation. Toxins will be moved and removed through sweating while you exercise. Before you begin any exercise regime, it is recommended that you consult a doctor or health practitioner.

When you begin to exercise, you may experience some symptoms as you start to detoxify that are not too pleasant. Apart from experiencing some sore muscles, as you begin to use ones you didn't know you had, you may experience a feeling of nausea, headaches, lethargy, mucous, cold- or flu-like symptoms, difficulty sleeping, cravings, diarrhoea, constipation, feeling of weakness, tiredness, gas, sneezing (especially in the morning when you wake), and foul-smelling sweat or urine.

You may experience some or none of these symptoms as toxins begin to move from your body, depending on how toxic your body is, and the route it is using to eliminate them. Do not let these symptoms deter you from starting an exercise routine. Exercise is a vital component in your journey to wellness, and is necessary if you want your skin and health to improve.

I recommend that you join a gym to get specialised advice and a personalised exercise program. At a minimum, do moderate exercise thirty minutes a day, three times a week. Please check with your health professional if you are of poor health, have heart problems, are obese, or have any other conditions that may inhibit exercise or put the body under undue stress. At the very least you can start walking for twenty minutes a day, three days a week.

It is vital that you drink adequate amounts of water during exercise. This will help your body detoxify and stay hydrated.

Epsom salt bath

I love to be in the water. It is very soothing to me on all levels, and I have an Epsom salt bath two or three times a week.

Soak in a bath with one cup of Epsom salts added to it and soak for twenty minutes. This will help remove toxins from you. Not only will this help draw toxins out of your skin, it will also infuse supplies of magnesium back into your body. Epsom salt contains magnesium sulphate, which is easily absorbed through the skin.

Magnesium is used for over three hundred biochemical reactions in the body. Epsom salt baths are also great to relieve stress, relieve pain, detoxify, and soothe you.

Chapter 17

Once You Start the Treatment

Once you begin taking the red clover combination supplements, your body will begin detoxifying and eliminating the old waste that is sitting in your cells. It is possible that your body may eliminate some of these toxins and waste through your skin *initially*; this may create more lesions or make the current lesions worse. Do not panic; this will be temporary and is referred to as a *healing crisis*. This is when, as conditions begin to get better, they may appear to be getting worse, but only for a short time. Once the supplements, diet, and lifestyle changes begin to support and enhance the function of your liver, bowel, and kidneys, you will begin to eliminate most of your waste successfully through them, rather than through your skin. If your skin gets worse, do not stop taking the red clover combination capsules. Continue their use and, fairly soon, you will see improvement again.

As your body begins detoxifying, you may find that you feel a bit unwell, develop cold-like symptoms, or experience headaches, runny nose, sneezing, tiredness, or other minor symptoms. These will pass in a few days. Just continue to adhere to the changes you have made to your diet and continue to take your supplements. Make sure that you drink lots of water to help your body eliminate this waste.

You may also find that you seem to have a lot of bowel movements; the faecal matter may be a mixture of colours and may smell very bad. This is due to the herbs in the red clover combination, and any extra fibre you are taking that is removing old waste from the bowel—this is good. If you are not having at least one bowel movement a day, you need to take a fibre supplement to encourage and promote bowel movements. The more waste that is eliminated through the bowel, the less waste may be eliminated through the skin. It is important that you concentrate on eating high-fibre foods, fruits, and vegetables, and get your bowel working regularly. Without doing this, you will slow down the healing of your skin.

Due to your increase in water intake, you may urinate more often and your urine may smell or be brownish in colour. For me, these signs were great as it meant that my body was beginning to work better and eliminate old waste.

Once I started taking the supplements, I noticed that the scales of skin on top of the lesions were thicker and were peeling off, which made them look worse. But as the layers of scale came off, I noticed that the lesions underneath were less red and not as raised up as they had been previously. The scale layer that was left was thinner, until there was barely a scaly layer at all. I then began to notice that in some lesions, the centre had small amounts of normal skin. They seemed to be healing from the centre out. My scalp began to heal first, and then I noticed other areas beginning to clear up and disappear.

I had to work hard to remember to take the supplements every day, and sometimes it felt like it was a lot to do, especially as I had also changed my diet, but I just kept reminding myself of my overall goal. My goal was to be able to have beautiful skin again, to be able to wear what I wanted, and to feel good. Those were such worthwhile goals that they kept me motivated to take my supplements, drink water, and resist foods that were not good for me. I constantly motivated myself by talking to myself, egging myself on, and providing internal encouragement, especially in the beginning before I could see any outward signs of improvement in my skin.

Some areas of skin responded very fast, while other areas responded quite slowly in comparison. The areas where the lesions had been for the shortest time seemed to heal the quickest—the ones caused by the streptococcus throat infection healed very rapidly, but the older plaque psoriasis areas took a bit longer.

One thing that amazes me is that, even where the lesions previously were, the skin is now completely normal. I have very few areas that are scarred, and those darkened areas are fading every day. For the most part, it was just a matter of getting a bit of a tan on the skin, as the areas that had previously had the psoriasis were completely white, whereas my skin is normally quite olive. The first summer, you could still see the difference in colour even after a tan, but this summer the skin tone is virtually even. I want to add that I was very careful and did not sit in the sun. I exposed myself to small amounts of sun every few days, and used a sunscreen to protect from burning.

For me, it doesn't matter if the skin tone does not even out completely, as I can easily cover it with one of the many skin-bronzing cosmetics on the market. The texture of my skin is now totally normal and can be easily coloured using a cosmetic. When I had psoriasis, I couldn't cover up because the lesions were raised and scaly. There was no way to make it appear normal, no matter how much product I applied. A skin bronzer is nothing compared to the joy of being able to bare my skin, feel normal, and know that no one is staring at awful-looking lesions all over my body.

I believe it is possible for you to have great skin, too. Use this as an opportunity for you to feel better about yourself. Don't look on the diet change and restrictions as a punishment, or feel like you are missing out. This is your opportunity to be well! Look on it as a challenge to get your body and skin well. Appreciate the changes you have made and the effort you have put in. Praise yourself, encourage yourself, and use old pictures of when you had good skin as motivation. If you've never had good skin, cut out a picture from a magazine of a body with good skin and attach your head to it. Hang these pictures up to remind yourself of why you are making these changes, and what you are going to achieve. Concentrate on your skin being beautiful, rather than being critical about how it currently looks.

Get a new hairstyle or buy some new clothes, encourage yourself to feel better and better about how you look. If you can't quite face buying new clothes yet, cut out pictures of the ones you are going to wear when your skin has cleared up. Put these pictures up on a board where you can see them. Allow yourself to think about how great it will be to have clear skin.

Reward yourself for doing so well and sticking to the supplement regime, and dietary and lifestyle changes. Take a vacation, go and see a movie, or have a dinner out. Reward yourself with something you like.

Chapter 18

How I Believe It Worked

I believe that taking the herbal combination and other supplements helped my body run better; because it was receiving extra nutrients, it was able to eliminate more waste (including old waste) via the bowel, kidneys, and liver, rather than through the skin. The digestive system was being supported to work better and extra enzymes were being taken to aid in digesting and assimilating the food I was eating. One of the main factors was that my liver was being stimulated and supported to work better and, therefore, my whole system was able to function more efficiently because this was helping with food absorption, toxin elimination, fat digestion, blood cleansing, and overall health. I was limiting the harmful and artificial ingredients in my diet and aiding the removal of waste by increasing my fibre intake, both through food choices and supplementation when necessary.

I know how easy it is to be depressed by this condition, and I know how hard it can be to help yourself when you are feeling depressed and have low self-esteem. Look inside yourself and know that you are worth the effort. This protocol worked for me and I am sure it will work for you.

I want you to understand why these supplements are necessary and what they do for you. I recommend that you do everything I suggest. This will ensure you get the best possible results in the least possible time. You may have a different form of psoriasis than mine, but by using all the treatments I suggest, you give yourself the best possible chance of beating this condition.

I also advise you to keep taking the red clover combination capsules after your skin condition has cleared up, or find an alternative supplement to keep your blood cleansed and bowel, liver, and kidneys working well. Get advice from your natural health specialist about your options, and which products may be best for you. I speak from experience, as my skin had almost completely cleared, with just a few spots left that were nearly gone, and I ran out of red clover combination capsules. I didn't refill my supply, believing that my body was functioning well by itself. I thought I was cured and didn't need the capsules anymore. I was wrong. Although my skin stayed stable for quite a while, before I knew it I had a fresh outbreak of lesions. I started back on the capsules and it took time before I could see the lesions begin to go away again. I believe that I will probably need to take these capsules or something similar, to keep my elimination system supported and working well for the rest of my life.

Section 5

What Supplements Do You Need to Take?

Chapter 19

A Guide on What to Take

I realise that it can all seem a bit confusing when you are attempting to work out what you need to take. Here is a sample questionnaire to help you assess which supplements may be right for you. Please consult a natural health professional before taking any regime of supplements, to ensure they don't aggravate any other current health problems and don't interfere or limit the actions of any medications you are currently taking. If you are unsure, seek professional medical advice.

CONSTIPATION

- Do you often sit on the toilet feeling like you have to have a bowel movement and nothing happens?
- Do you strain to expel a bowel movement?
- Do you have a full feeling even after you have just been to the toilet?
- Do you have days where you do not have a bowel movement?
- Do you have abdominal discomfort or pain?

If you answered yes to any of these questions, you are probably constipated and need to increase your dietary fibre and water intake and take a fibre supplement, which will help clear the bowel and get you regular again.

DEHYDRATION

- Do you drink mostly fizzy or caffeinated drinks?
- Do you drink more than three cups of coffee a day?
- Does your urine appear dark yellow?
- Do you drink less than eight cups of plain water a day?
- Do you have dry lips?

If you answered yes to any of these questions, then you need to drink more water.

MULTI-VITAMIN SUPPLEMENTS

- Do you have cracks in the corners of your mouth?
- Do you eat a lot of fast food and processed foods?
- Do you feel tired and worn out all the time, even when you just wake up?
- Does most of the food you eat come from boxes or packets?
- Do you feel sluggish, both mentally and physically?
- Do you get overwhelmed by stress or depression?
- Does your hair look limp and unhealthy?
- Do you get sick or feel unwell often?
- Have you been anaemic?
- Does your skin look dull and unhealthy?

If you answered yes to more than one of these questions, you may need to take a multi-vitamin supplement to provide adequate nutrients to support the body to function correctly. Consult a natural health professional for advice on a quality, highly absorbable multi-vitamin supplement that will suit your age, lifestyle, and nutritional requirements.

DIGESTION

- Do you burp a lot while eating?
- Do you feel full for hours after eating?

- Do you notice undigested food particles in your faeces?
- Do you eat mostly well-done cooked foods?
- Do you have abdominal pains?
- Do you pass a lot of wind?

If you answered yes to any of these questions, you may benefit from taking digestive enzymes with your meals.

How to choose a good digestive enzyme supplement
Different food groups require different enzymes to digest them. Choose a broad-spectrum digestive enzyme supplement containing different enzymes, to ensure maximum digestive support. A typical Western meal will require protease, amylase, lipase, sucrose, cellulose, and lactase enzymes to digest it. If you are unsure, ask the advice of a natural health specialist at your local store to get the right digestive enzyme for you.

BOWEL BACTERIA

- Do you pass wind a lot?
- Do you often feel bloated?
- Do your faeces smell bad?
- Do you take or have you taken the contraceptive pill?
- Have you ever taken antibiotics?
- Do you eat a diet high in sugar and sugary foods including fizzy drinks?

If you answered yes to any of these questions, you will need a course of probiotics. I recommend everyone takes at least one course per year.

To choose a good probiotic, look for one that:

- Is made by a reputable company
- Is coated to survive digestion and get through to the bowel
- Is not very cheap; often price is an indicator of quality

- Contains bacteria from the lactobacillus and bifidobacterium family
- Contains at least 10 million bacteria per capsule
- Guarantees it contains live bacteria

If you are in doubt of which one to choose, consult a natural health professional at your local health store; they will help you to choose a quality probiotic suitable for you.

ZINC DEFICIENCY

- Do you suffer from constant colds or infections?
- Do your wounds heal slowly?
- Have you lost your sense of taste?
- Is your appetite poor?
- Do you have white marks on your fingernails?
- Does your skin look unhealthy?

If you answered yes to any of the above questions, you probably have a zinc deficiency. Your skin condition alone can indicate a deficiency. Get a zinc taste test done to identify how high your need for zinc is. Go to a natural health care professional, naturopath, or health food shop for professional advice on the best type of zinc for you. If you are extremely zinc deficient, you may need a supplement in a liquid form because your digestive system may not be able to absorb zinc efficiently, and the liquid form will make it easier for your body to assimilate it.

OMEGA-3 OILS

- Do you eat oily fish three times a week (e.g., salmon, herring, etc.)?
- Do you eat soybeans, tofu, or other beans three times a week?
- Do you use grape seed oil or flaxseed oil daily? (raw)
- If you have answered yes to these questions you may not need

omega supplementation. If you find that your skin is still very dry and scaly after a month of taking the other supplements, consider short-term supplementation of an omega-3 supplement.

If you answered no to more than one of these questions, then you will probably need an omega-3 supplement.

FLOWER ESSENCES

- Are you often overwhelmed by stress?
- Do you often feel depressed or blue for no apparent reason?
- Do you overreact to problems?
- Do your emotions jump from happiness to sadness quickly?
- Do you feel emotionally exhausted?
- Do you feel like you need emotional support?

We all need emotional support at some times in our lives; flower essences are a fantastic remedy to help emotionally support you. They can be custom made to suit your current emotional status or problems. You can also buy Rescue Remedy® and use this any time you get really stressed. I definitely recommend using flower essences to help cope with the stresses of modern living; they will also help you to cope with the stress of changing your lifestyle and diet.

You can purchase Rescue Remedy® at all good health shops and pharmacies. You can also find trained practitioners who will mix you a custom blend of flower essences to suit your particular needs.

CHECKLIST OF SUPPLEMENTS

The red clover combination supplement is necessary; do not run out of this, and keep taking it.

The zinc taste test should be done to check for zinc deficiency, as zinc is responsible for skin health.

I recommend that everyone takes at least one course of probiotics; this ensures that your bowel will have a good supply of good bacteria and may help your body assimilate nutrients correctly.

Tick the supplements you need to take:

- ☐ Red clover combination
- ☐ Zinc taste test and possible supplementation if needed
- ☐ Probiotics—at least a one month course every year
- ☐ Fibre for constipation
- ☐ Multi-vitamin supplement
- ☐ Omega-3 oils
- ☐ Digestive enzymes with every meal
- ☐ Flower essences

Printed in July 2019
by Rotomail Italia S.p.A., Vignate (MI) - Italy